ON CALL

PROCEDURES

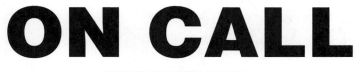

D0325219

STEPHEN D. BRES

Assistant Professor of Surgery
Division of Plastic and Reconstructive Surgery
University of Southern California School of Medicine
Attending Plastic Surgeon
Children's Hospital
Los Angeles, California

□ □ □

GREGG A. ADAMS, MD

Staff Surgeon
Santa Clara Valley Medical Center
San Jose, California

Clinical Instructor
Department of General Surgery
Stanford University Medical Center
Stanford, California

W.B. SAUNDERS COMPANY
A Harcourt Health Sciences Company
Philadelphia London New York St. Louis Sydney Toronto

W.B. SAUNDERS COMPANY
A Harcourt Health Sciences Company

The Curtis Center
Independence Square West
Philadelphia, Pennsylvania 19106

Library of Congress Cataloging-in-Publication Data

Bresnick, Stephen D.
On call procedures / Stephen D. Bresnick, Gregg A. Adams.—1st ed.

p.   cm.

Includes index.

ISBN 0–7216–7304–X

1. Surgical emergencies—Handbooks, manuals, etc.   2. Hospitals–
    Medical staff—Handbooks, manuals, etc.   I. Adams, Gregg A.
    II. Title. [DNLM: 1. Emergency handbooks.   2. Surgical Procedures,
    Operative handbooks.   WO 39 B842o 2000]

RD93.B69 2000   617.'026—dc21

DNLM/DLC   98-19200

Acquisitions Editor: William Schmitt
Project Manager: Amy Norwitz
Illustration Specialist: Peg Shaw

ON CALL PROCEDURES   ISBN 0–7216–7304–X

Printed in the United States of America.

Last digit is the print number: 9   8   7   6   5   4   3   2   1

PREFACE

The delivery of medical care to hospitalized patients is an orchestration of disciplines. Knowledge of pharmacology, anatomy, and disease pathophysiology needs to be applied to the specific circumstances of individual patients. Each treatment regimen, no matter how well conceived, may be altered by unanticipated changes in patient condition, interactions of medications, and complications of procedures.

The tools of medicine are complex and various. Therapy may include patient education, administration of medication, surgical intervention, and other modalities. Many individuals with various specialized skills and knowledge are required to help a patient negotiate a disease course. While a multidisciplinary approach is desirable and possible during the light of day, a physician on call at night generally has fewer resources readily available.

Often, the management of patients requires invasive procedures for diagnosis or treatment. The rapid and appropriate application of these techniques is required to ensure effective patient care. While many procedures are straightforward in description, they require practice and repetition to be performed safely.

On Call Procedures is designed to give the on-call physician and the physician-in-training some of the basic tools required to care for patients in the middle of the night. It gives indications and step-by-step instructions for a variety of medical and surgical procedures. Also described are some of the more common complications and problems encountered with these procedures. *On Call Procedures* is a concise, helpful guide to the safe and effective application of medical techniques. Together with the "pearls" given by the attending physician while on rounds, and the tips offered by a chief resident over your shoulder during a procedure, this book will supply the needed information and confidence to approach a variety of on-call situations.

Stephen D. Bresnick

Gregg A. Adams

STRUCTURE OF THE BOOK

This book is designed to give the reader step-by-step instructions for the performance of many routine bedside medical procedures. Each section is introduced, and the procedures are described in general terms. The indications and precautions for the procedure are delineated. The book then gives detailed instructions complete with appropriate technical details and numerous detailed illustrations of anatomy. Lastly, some of the commonly encountered problems with placement, maintenance, or removal of medical applications are discussed.

INTRODUCTION

Time spent on call is often stressful and busy. At night, there may be fewer staff members available for immediate consultation and often little time for learning new or perfecting infrequently used procedures. However, patients may benefit from the swift and sure action of an on-call team member who is able to perform a lifesaving or care-facilitating procedure.

Like all techniques, those described in this book will take some practice to perfect. Some individuals may perform a procedure for the first time using these easy-to-follow steps, and others will improve their technique using some of the steps described. Even the most experienced operator may benefit from a periodic review of the anatomy described herein.

COMMONLY USED ABBREVIATIONS

ABCs	airway, breathing, circulation (first steps of evaluating a critically ill patient)
ABG	arterial blood gas
ACE	angiotensin-converting enzyme
AF	atrial fibrillation
AIDS	acquired immunodeficiency syndrome
ant	anterior
Ao	aorta
AP	anterior-to-posterior direction (as in path of x-rays)
AV	atrioventricular
AZT	zidovudine
B	bilateral
BID	twice daily
BP	blood pressure
bpm	beats per minute
BS	breath sounds
°C	degrees Celsius
C & S	culture and sensitivity
Ca$^+$	calcium ion
CBC	complete blood count
cc	cubic centimeter (milliliter)
CCU	critical care unit
CHF	congestive heart failure
Cl$^-$	chloride ion
cm	centimeter
cm H$_2$O	centimeters of water
CNS	central nervous system
CO$_2$	carbon dioxide

COPD	chronic obstructive pulmonary disease
CPB	cardiopulmonary bypass
CPP	cranial perfusion pressure (MAP − ICP)
CPR	cardiopulmonary resuscitation
CT	computed tomography
CVA	cerebrovascular accident (stroke)
CVP	central venous pressure
CXR	chest x-ray
DBP	diastolic blood pressure
DIC	disseminated intravascular coagulation
DVT	deep venous thrombosis
Dx	diagnosis
ECG	electrocardiogram
EMD	electromechanical dissociation (PEA)
ET	endotracheal
°F	degrees Fahrenheit
Fio$_2$	fraction of oxygen in inspired air
Fr	French
g	gram
GI	gastrointestinal
Hb	hemoglobin
HCO$_3$	bicarbonate ion
Hct	hematocrit
HIV	human immunodeficiency virus
HR	heart rate
HTN	hypertension
Hx	history
IABP	intra-aortic balloon pump
ICP	intracranial pressure
ICU	intensive care unit
IJ	internal jugular vein (or line)
IM	intramuscular

inf	inferior
I/O	intake and output measurements
IP	intraperitoneal
IU	international unit
IV	intravenous
IVC	inferior vena cava
J	joule
JVD	jugular venous distention
K+	potassium ion
kg	kilogram
KUB	"kidney, ureter, bladder," a flat-plate radiograph of the abdomen
L	liter
L	left side
lat	lateral
LDH	lactate dehydrogenase
LP	lumbar puncture
LR	lactated Ringer's solution
MAP	mean arterial pressure
med	medial
mEq	milliequivalent
mg	milligram
μg	microgram
Mg+	magnesium ion
MI	myocardial infarction
ml	milliliter
mm	millimeter
mm³	cubic millimeter
mm Hg	millimeters of mercury
mmol	millimolar concentration
mOsm	milliosmolar concentration

MRI	magnetic resonance imaging
MSO$_4$	morphine sulfate
Na$^+$	sodium ion
NAVELS	nerve→artery→vein→empty space→lymphatics→symphysis pubis
NG	nasogastric
NPO	*nil per os,* nothing by mouth
NS	normal saline
NSAID	nonsteroidal anti-inflammatory drug
O$_2$	oxygen
OR	operating room
P	pulse rate
PA	posterior-to-anterior direction (as in path of x-rays)
PAC	premature atrial contraction
PaO$_2$	alveolar partial pressure of oxygen
Pao$_2$	arterial partial pressure of oxygen
P[A-a]O$_2$	alveolar-arterial oxygen gradient
PAR	"procedure, alternatives, risk," used with surgical informed consent
Pco$_2$	partial pressure of carbon dioxide
PCWP	pulmonary capillary wedge pressure
PEA	pulseless electrical activity (EMD)
pH	$(-)$ log of hydrogen ion concentration
PICC	peripherally inserted central catheter
plt	platelet count
PO	*per os*, by mouth
post	posterior
PR	per rectum
PRN	*pro re nata*, as necessary
PSVT	paroxysmal supraventricular tachycardia
PT	prothrombin time
PTT	partial thromboplastin time
PVC	premature ventricular contraction

PVR	pulmonary vascular resistance
QD	every day
QHS	at bedtime
QID	four times daily
R	right side
RBC	red blood cell
resp	respiratory
RN	registered nurse
R/O	rule out
RR	respiratory rate
Rx	prescription
Sao$_2$	oxygen saturation of arterial blood
SBP	systolic blood pressure
SL	sublingual
SLE	systemic lupus erythematosus
SOB	short of breath, shortness of breath
SQ	subcutaneous
sup	superior
SV	stroke volume
Svo$_2$	oxygen saturation of venous blood
SVC	superior vena cava
SVR	systemic vascular resistance
T	temperature
TB	tuberculosis
TCP	transcutaneous pacing
TID	three times daily
tPA	tissue plasminogen activator
TPN	total parenteral nutrition
TPVR	total peripheral vascular resistance
Tx	treatment
UA	urinalysis
UO	urine output

US	ultrasound
VC	vena cava
VF	ventricular fibrillation
VS	vital signs
VT	ventricular tachycardia
WBC	white blood cell
wt	weight

CONTENTS

APPENDICES

GENERAL CONSIDERATIONS

THE NEED FOR MEDICAL PROCEDURES

The care of patients in the hospital involves the coordination of many disciplines. The technology of medicine has advanced such that the function of many organ systems may be directly monitored and manipulated. To achieve this, invasive procedures often are necessary to place lines, drain fluid collections, or facilitate monitoring.

Any invasive procedure has risks as well as benefits, and a knowledge of these will temper the use of these techniques. To safely implement these technologies, it is necessary to be versed in the placement and care of the lines or tubes and to be able to handle the potential complications of their placement and use.

Most invasive procedures will require informed consent before they are started. Be sure the procedure is explained to the patient by someone who is familiar with the risks and complications. A signed consent form should be obtained before the administration of sedative medication and should be in the medical record before the procedure is begun.

DOCUMENTATION OF PROCEDURES

Medical documentation is not just a medicolegal issue; it also is a primary form of communication between team members. Invasive procedures must be documented as a procedure note in the chart; an example of a procedure note is given in Figure 2–1. Be sure to list which medications were administered and what monitoring was used. In addition, legibly write your name and beeper number next to your signature. Make sure your plan is well spelled out, so that if you are relying on someone else to follow the patient or remove sutures, that person will know exactly what to do. When it is appropriate, a diagram is helpful to aid in the care of a tube or line. Often, an invasive procedure

Indication:	Left malignant pleural effusion
Procedure:	Placement of left chest tube
Staff:	Dr. Bresnick (in attendance)
Assistant:	Dr. Adams
Sedation:	Midazolam 2 mg IV and morphine sulfate 5 mg IV
Anesthesia:	1% Lidocaine local 5 ml SQ
Monitoring:	Continuous pulse oximetry, oxygen 2 L nasal cannula
Procedure notes:	28 Fr straight chest tube placed by trochar from fourth interspace midaxillary line to posterior basal position; 500 ml of straw-colored fluid removed; attached to Pleurovac to 20 cm H_2O suction
Cultures:	Gram stain, aerobic and anaerobic cultures, AFB, and fungal cultures
Special studies:	Cell count and differential, cytospin for cytology, and LDH, protein
Blood loss:	5 ml
CXR:	Good placement of the tube, no pneumothorax noted
Complications:	None; patient tolerated procedure well
Follow-up:	We will follow with the primary team and plan for chemical pleurodesis in the future, if indicated

Figure 2–1 □ Example of a procedural note. Remember to sign and date the note. Indicate the time that the procedure was performed, and include your beeper or phone number.

will need to be performed on a patient who has a different primary care team. It is even more important to document your procedures well so that there is no confusion as to what has been done and how to take care of the results. It is important to document the indication for the procedure.

HAZARDS OF BODY FLUID EXPOSURE

The practice of medicine has inherent risks. The exposure to blood and secretion-borne disease is significant and should always be considered. Specifically, the transmission of human immunodeficiency virus or hepatitis virus to a health care provider from an infected patient, although infrequent, is always a real risk. Precautions must *always* be taken, especially with patients for whom you have no first-hand knowledge (Table 3–1).

If blood contact does occur, find out hospital policies regarding the treatment of significant blood-borne exposures. Know where to seek first aid as required. Ensure that tetanus and hepatitis B vaccinations are up to date (Table 3–2).

Table 3–1 □ UNIVERSAL PRECAUTIONS TO PREVENT TRANSMISSION OF HUMAN IMMUNODEFICIENCY VIRUS

Universal Precautions

Because a medical history and physical examination cannot reliably identify all patients infected with human immunodeficiency virus (HIV) or other blood-borne pathogens, blood and body fluid precautions should be consistently used for all patients, especially those in emergency care settings in which the risk of blood exposure is increased and the infection status of the patient is usually not known.

1. Use appropriate barrier protection to prevent skin and mucous membrane exposure when exposure to blood, body fluids containing blood, or other body fluids to which universal precautions apply (see below) is anticipated. Wear gloves when touching blood or body fluids, mucous membranes, or nonintact skin of all patients; when handling items or surfaces soiled with blood of body fluids; and when performing venipuncture and other vascular access procedures. Change gloves after contact with each patient; do not wash or disinfect gloves for reuse. Wear masks and protective eyewear or face shields during procedures that are likely to generate droplets of blood or other body fluids to prevent exposure of mucous membranes of the mouth, nose, and eyes. Wear gowns or aprons during procedures that are likely to generate splashes of blood or other body fluids.

2. Wash hands and other skin surfaces immediately and thoroughly following contaminations with blood, body fluids containing blood, or other body fluids to which universal precautions apply. Wash hands immediately after gloves are removed.

Table 3–1 □ UNIVERSAL PRECAUTIONS TO PREVENT TRANSMISSION OF HUMAN IMMUNODEFICIENCY VIRUS *Continued*

Universal Precautions *Continued*

3. Take care to prevent injuries when using needles, scalpels, and other sharp instruments or devices, when handling sharp instruments after procedures, when cleaning used instruments, and when disposing of used needles. Do not recap needles by hand; do not remove used needles from disposable syringes by hand; and do not bend, break, or otherwise manipulate used needles by hand. Place used disposable syringes and needles, scalpel blades, and other sharp items in puncture-resistant disposal containers, which should be located as close to the use area as is practical.
4. Although saliva has not been implicated in HIV transmission, the need for emergency mouth-to-mouth resuscitation should be minimized by making mouthpieces, resuscitation bags, or other ventilation devices available for use in areas in which the need for resuscitation is predictable.
5. Health care workers with exudative lesions or weeping dermatitis should refrain from all direct patient care and from handling patient care equipment until the condition resolves.

Universal precautions are intended to supplement rather than replace recommendations for routine infection control, such as hand washing and use of gloves to prevent gross microbial contamination of hands. In addition, implementation of universal precautions does not eliminate the need for other category of disease-specific isolation precautions, such as enteric precautions for infectious diarrhea of isolation for pulmonary tuberculosis. Universal precautions are not intended to change waste management programs undertaken in accordance with state and local regulations.

Body Fluids to Which Universal Precautions Apply

Universal precautions apply to blood and other body fluids containing visible blood. Blood is the single most important source of HIV, hepatitis B or C virus, and other blood-borne pathogens in the occupational setting. Universal precautions also apply to tissues, semen, vaginal secretions, and the following fluids: cerebrospinal, synovial, pleural, peritoneal, and amniotic.

Universal precautions do not apply to feces, nasal secretions, sputum, sweat, tears, urine, and vomitus unless they contain visible blood. Universal precautions also do not apply to human breast milk, although gloves may be worn by health care workers in situations in which exposure to breast milk might be frequent. In addition, universal precautions do not apply to saliva. Gloves need not be worn when feeding patients or wiping saliva from skin, although special precautions are recommended for dentistry, in which contamination of saliva with blood is predictable. The risk of transmission of HIV, as well as hepatitis B or C virus, from these fluids and materials is extremely low or nonexistent.

Table continued on following page

Table 3–1 □ UNIVERSAL PRECAUTIONS TO PREVENT TRANSMISSION OF HUMAN IMMUNODEFICIENCY VIRUS *Continued*

Use of Gloves for Phlebotomy

Gloves should be effective in reducing the incidence of blood contamination of hands during phlebotomy (drawing of blood samples), but they cannot prevent penetrating injuries caused by needles or other sharp instruments. In universal precautions, all blood is assumed to be potentially infectious for blood-borne pathogens. Some institutions have relaxed recommendations for the use of gloves for the phlebotomy by skilled health care workers in settings in which the prevalence of blood-borne pathogens is known to be very low (e.g., volunteer blood donation centers). Institutions that judge that routine use of gloves for all phlebotomies is not necessary should periodically reevaluate their policy. Gloves should always be available for those who wish to use them for phlebotomy. In addition, the following general guidelines apply:

1. Use gloves for performing phlebotomy if cuts, scratches, or other breaks in the skin are present.
2. Use gloves in situations in which contamination with blood may occur—for example, when performing phlebotomy on an uncooperative patient.
3. Use gloves for performing finger or heel sticks on infants and children.
4. Use gloves when training persons to do phlebotomies.

From Scientific American Medicine, Section 7, Subsection XI. © 1990 Scientific American, Inc. All rights reserved.

Table 3–2 □ FIRST AID FOLLOWING BLOOD OR BODY FLUID EXPOSURES (DO NOT DELAY!)

1. Immediately clean the exposed site. For skin sites, wash with detergent and water or a 1:10 bleach solution. For eyes and other mucous membranes, use saline or water. Wash for 5 minutes.
2. Save the instrument in a sharps container for testing later.
3. Seek out a supervisor for instructions. A specific protocol may be in place for your institution.
4. Most likely, blood for serology testing will be drawn from you and the patient from whom the fluid originated.
5. Ensure tetanus and HBV vaccinations are up to date.
6. Some institutions recommend AZT (zidovudine) prophylaxis.

CONSCIOUS SEDATION

Some on-call procedures will require conscious sedation. Invasive procedures in awake and alert patients may be painful and anxiety provoking. It is appropriate to give sedation to stable patients whose vital signs (VS) are monitored. The primary objectives of conscious sedation are patient comfort and safety. In this chapter, the indications, techniques, and pitfalls of conscious sedation are discussed.

■ INDICATIONS

Conscious sedation is best used when performing anxiety-provoking or painful procedures, and it is most often used in conjunction with local anesthesia. For example, chest tube thoracostomy in awake and alert patients is best performed with local anesthesia supplemented by conscious sedation. On the other hand, a critically ill and unstable patient is best treated with tube thoracostomy with local anesthesia alone. Remember that most sedatives are respiratory and cardiovascular depressants, and the risks associated with giving these drugs must be weighed against the benefits.

Always be a humane physician. The appropriate use of conscious sedation techniques is humane and will be appreciated by the patient. Consider the use of conscious sedation in conjunction with local anesthesia if the administration is safe, the patient is well monitored, and you feel confident with the techniques outlined in this chapter. Many hospitals have protocols that outline appropriate monitoring and care of a patient during conscious sedation.

■ CONTRAINDICATIONS

Avoid the use of conscious sedation in situations in which it may be unsafe. The following scenarios would not be appropriate for administration of conscious sedation.

1. Patients with hypotension, respiratory sedation, or labile vital signs
2. Uncooperative patients
3. Patients with obtunded protective reflexes
4. Patients with known sensitivity to sedatives
5. Patients who cannot be monitored adequately or in whom there is no IV access

6. Situations in which reversal drugs (e.g., naloxone hydrochloride [Narcan]) are not available

■ PRECAUTIONS

Always be alert for the major side effects of conscious sedation.
- Respiratory depression
- Loss of airway
- Cardiovascular depression

Also, consider the following useful guides in determining drug dosing and patient fragility.
- Patient age: Elderly patients have lower organ system reserves and may require lower doses of sedative medication.
- Preoperative anxiety level: Very anxious patients may require higher drug doses, yet sedatives should always be titrated.
- If possible, obtain a history of previous problems with sedation.
- Beware of patients with cardiac or pulmonary disease; these patients may best be sedated in the operating room (OR) by an anesthesiologist.

■ EQUIPMENT NEEDED

1. Adequate IV access
2. Oxygen saturation (SaO_2) monitor
3. Blood pressure (BP) cuff or functional arterial line
4. Stethoscope
5. Oxygen (O_2) availability, mask, O_2 tubing
6. Appropriate sedatives and their antagonist-reversal agents
7. Know the location of resuscitative equipment

■ TECHNIQUE

1. Review the patient's medical history, VS, and any known sensitivity or allergy to sedative-hypnotics.
2. Obtain an informed consent prior to administration of sedative medications.
3. Clinically assess the patient.
   Evaluate mental status, body weight, fragility, and patient age. Also look at the patient's respiratory pattern, rate, tidal volume, and airway patency.
4. Obtain preprocedure VS.
5. Ask for an RN or another physician to help you monitor the patient. Follow established guidelines for your institution.

6. Place O_2 tubing on the patient, and attach and activate an SaO_2 monitor.
7. Ensure that SaO_2 is appropriate before giving sedatives.
8. Slowly administer increments of sedatives. Always titrate to effect. Keep in mind
   a. A darkened room helps make sedation easier as long as you have the light for any necessary procedure.
   b. Talk to the patient while administering a sedative.
      When speech becomes slurred or when a normal SaO_2 level begins to drop (100% becomes 94% to 95%), the patient should be sufficiently sedated to make the procedure more tolerable.
   c. Consider starting with either a narcotic or benzodiazepine.
      Choose short-acting drugs over longer-acting drugs. Synergistic effects are achieved when narcotics are combined with benzodiazepines.
   d. Midazolam (Versed) is an ideal sedative.
      It has a short half-life and gives an amnesiac effect. Start with 0.5 mg and titrate to effect with 0.5-mg increments. It is important to start with low doses because some patients are sensitive to benzodiazepines. Other benzodiazepines are available, but they have longer half-lives. Midazolam alone may provide adequate sedation (Table 4–1).
   e. You may want to administer a subsedative dose of midazolam or other benzodiazepine and supplement it with a narcotic.
      This has the advantage of adding pain receptor blockade (narcotic blockade) to the sedative cocktail. You can use morphine (1- to 2-mg IV increments, up to 10 mg), meperidine (Demerol; 15 to 20-mg IV increments, up to 100 mg), or fentanyl (Sublimaze; 0.05- to 0.1-mg IV increments, up to

Table 4–1 □ COMMON BENZODIAZEPINES USEFUL IN SEDATION AND THEIR ANTAGONIST

Drug	Dose and Duration
Agonists	
Midazolam (Versed)	0.5–1-mg increments IV, up to 10 mg; 1–2-hr duration
Diazepam (Valium)	1–2-mg increments IV, up to 10 mg; 4–6-hr duration
Antagonist	
Flumazenil (Romazicon)	0.2 mg IV over 15 seconds; repeat as necessary in increments of 0.2 mg every 60 seconds, to a maximum dose of 1 mg

Table 4–2 □ **COMMON NARCOTICS USEFUL IN SEDATION**

Drug	Dose and Duration
Agonists	
Morphine sulfate	0.1–0.2 mg/kg, 1–3-mg increments, up to 10 mg; the "gold standard"; 2–4-hr duration
Fentanyl citrate (Sublimaze)	2–3 μg/kg, 50–100-μg increments, up to 500 μg; short-duration IV, very effective; 1–2-hr duration
Meperidine hydrochloride (Demerol)	25-mg increments IV, up to 100 mg; 2–4-hr duration
Antagonist	
Naloxone hydrochloride (Narcan)	0.2–2.0 mg IV/IM/SC every 5 minutes as necessary to a maximum dose of 10 mg

0.5 mg). Be aware of the risks and benefits of each narcotic. Always titrate to effect. Never give large bolus doses (Table 4–2).

f. In case a reversal of sedation is needed, always have at the bedside both a narcotic antagonist (naloxone hydrochloride, 0.2 to 2.0 mg IV/IM/SQ, repeat every 5 minutes as needed to a maximum dose of 10 mg) and a benzodiazepine antagonist (flumazenil [Romazicon], 0.2 mg IV administered over 15 seconds, repeat every 60 seconds as needed to a maximum dose of 1 mg). See also Tables 4–1 and 4–2.

9. After sedatives are administered
   a. Keep in verbal contact with the patient.
      You should not have a patient who is unresponsive to verbal stimuli. You are trying to achieve conscious sedation, not unconscious sedation.
   b. Check the VS and SaO_2 every 5 minutes for 30 minutes and then on a PRN basis. Follow existing guidelines.
   c. Concurrent with BP checks, evaluate pulse intensity, rate, and regularity.

■ **COMPLICATIONS/PROBLEMS**

1. Respiratory depression
   This is a significant and common problem that can occur during attempts to provide adequate sedation. This is best treated with the administration of a narcotic antagonist, benzodiazepine antagonist, or both (see 8.f, above).

2. Loss of airway

The airway may become obstructed during sedation procedures. If airway loss occurs, first reestablish the airway, and then administer sedative-reversal drugs as described earlier. Airway obstruction usually is caused by tongue and pharyngeal muscle relaxation due to the sedatives. The base of the tongue may fall to the back of the throat and obstruct the airway. This can be corrected by thrusting the lower jaw forward and placing forward pressure behind the mandibular angle/ramus region. A forward chin thrust also can help bring the tongue forward. It may be necessary to place an oral airway. Use a mask and a pressure bag to ventilate the patient if needed. Intubation may be required.

3. Aspiration

Conscious sedation should be induced only in patients who have had nothing by mouth (NPO) for 6 hours or longer. Sedation decreases airway control, and a patient who vomits is at risk of aspiration. Always be aware of the risk of aspiration, and do not sedate patients who have recently eaten.

4. Hypotension

Some patient may vasodilate in response to sedatives. These patients may become hypotensive. If this occurs, consider administering a normal saline (NS) fluid bolus to the patient, and concurrently administer reversal drugs. Most patients will rapidly respond to this treatment.

5

STERILE TECHNIQUE

In many procedures, it is imperative that sterile technique be observed. Although most sterile techniques are performed in a controlled fashion in the operating room (OR), the procedures described here may be done at the bedside and require special care to maintain sterility. The preparation and maintenance of a sterile field represent a skill that, once acquired, will be second-nature. For those new to surgery or the infrequent user of sterile techniques, here are a few tips:

1. **Prepare your environment.**
   Make sure that your work space is well lit and comfortable. Place the bed at a comfortable height, have the bedrails down, and get a chair if appropriate. Sterility is often broken by having to reposition lighting or draping. Clear the area of objects that might catch your sleeves or your feet. Have room to move.

2. **Make sure that all the instruments are available.**
   Anticipate what supplies and instruments you will need. Have them opened and within easy reach. This requires planning, but it will soon become routine.

3. **Have help standing by, if necessary.**
   You will need an extra pair of hands in many cases; make sure it is someone who is familiar with sterile technique. If you need more senior supervision, give that individual plenty of notice.

4. **Know the steps of the procedure.**
   Do a mental walk-through of the procedure before you put on your gloves. Check to ensure that the equipment needed for each step is available. It often is possible to line up the instruments in the order in which they are needed.

5. **Inform the patient that a sterile field is going to be used.**
   Instruct the patient not to touch areas of sterility. It also is important to reassure the patient if the drapes are going to temporarily cover the eyes or airway. Always explain if there are uncomfortable or painful steps in the process, and warn the patient before the pain. Sterility often is broken when a patient jumps after a painful stimulus such as a needlestick.

6. **Position the patient.**
   Place the patient in the position in which you want him or her, ensuring that any towel rolls are in place before beginning. The nurses will appreciate if you place a pad or diaper

under the region of the body that is to be prepped to protect the bed from drips of blood or soap.

7. **Prepare the insertion site.**

   Use an alcohol- or iodine-based disinfectant soap, and clean (or "prep") the area well. Solution on a gauze or prepackaged swab sticks may be used. Start from the center of the desired field and work your way outward, cleaning a wider area than you think necessary. Repeat with a fresh gauze or swab for a total of three cleanings. If desired, more than one area may be initially prepared. The second site may be kept sterile with a drape while the first site is being used.

8. **Scrub your hands with a disinfectant soap.**

   Remove rings and jewelry first. Put on a mask and cap before scrubbing, especially if the patient is immunocompromised or if an invasive line will be needed for a long time.

9. **Put on sterile gloves and gown.**

   Get help if you do not know how to do this in a sterile fashion.

10. **Drape the area with sterile towels.**

    Ensure that the only thing visible through the "window" made with the towels is "prepared" skin. The towel may come fenestrated, or a window may be made using two or more towels. The drapes may be held in place with towel clamps if desired.

11. **Try not to move from the sterile field unless absolutely necessary.**

    Once in place and working, be mindful of the nonsterile areas of your body (elbows, hair, waist).

12. **Work quickly but carefully.**

13. **Admit easily if there has been a break in sterility.**

    The constraints of time and pride may tempt you to overlook a minor break in sterility, but any time saved here will be more than taken up by the time required to care for a sicker patient if a complication arises. Do not hesitate to "break scrub," rewash, redrape, and begin again if you think that you compromised sterility. Do not put the patient at risk.

14. **The procedure is not done until the line is secured.**

    Secure the line or tube by taping, suturing, or tying down. Do this before removing the drapes. Make sure the line is secure even if a chest x-ray (CXR) is required to assess placement of the line before its use. You do not want your well-placed line to be dislodged during the confirmatory x-ray or while repositioning the patient.

15. **Protect the sterility of the line.**

    Place a dressing over the site, including an antimicrobial ointment. Confirm all connections and joints before careful removal of the drapes.

16. **"Reprep" and drape the area if repositioning of the line is necessary.**

    The cleansing of the area is no less vigorous if the line must be repositioned.

17. **When the procedure is completed, clean the area of soap.**

    The soaps used often are very irritating, so protect the skin by cleaning away the irritant.

18. **Be responsible for your own "sharps" disposal.**

    Do not leave this job to a nurse or student.

PROCEDURES

6

CRICOTHYROIDOTOMY

Cricothyroidotomy is an emergency procedure used for glottic or supraglottic airway obstruction. Second to orotracheal intubation, cricothyroidotomy is one of the fastest means of establishing an airway. This procedure should be reserved for when an airway is rapidly needed and less invasive attempts at establishing an airway have failed.

This procedure can be performed with the percutaneous placement of a large-bore needle through the cricothyroid membrane. However, a large-bore needle airway is tenuous, very small, and often inadequate. The formal, surgical cricothyroidotomy technique is described here.

■ INDICATIONS

1. Airway obstruction above the level of the cricoid cartilage
   It is important to keep in mind that this technique is useful only if the airway is patent below the cricoid cartilage. If obstruction is present inferior to the cricoid, cricothyroidotomy will not establish a patent airway.
2. Attempts to intubate that have failed, an airway that cannot be obtained by any other means, and a patient's life in jeopardy
3. Laryngeal trauma, mass, or hematoma with emergent need for airway

■ CONTRAINDICATIONS

1. Subglottic airway obstruction
   Cricothyroidotomy will be superior to the level of the obstruction, and airway patency will not be achieved.
2. Injudicious use
   This procedure should not be used in an on-call setting outside of emergency circumstances. Cricothyroidotomy is associated with potential complications more prevalent than intubation by a skilled operator.

3. Coagulopathy

Carefully consider the consequences of an invasive procedure such as cricothyroidotomy, and reserve its use for life-threatening situations. In coagulopathic patients, platelets, fresh frozen plasma, and other blood products may be needed to control postprocedure bleeding.

■ PRECAUTIONS

1. Know the regional anatomy.

It is critical to know the location of the cricothyroid membrane and the important structures adjacent to it (Fig. 6–1).
2. Use sterile technique if possible.

■ EQUIPMENT NEEDED

1. Adequate lighting
2. Suction
3. Local anesthesia if the patient is awake

Consider the use of 1% lidocaine with 1:100,000 epinephrine to help minimize cutaneous bleeding.

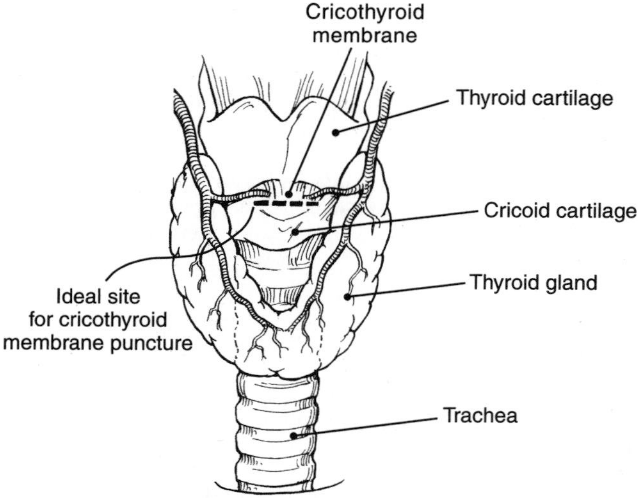

Figure 6–1 □ Anatomy of laryngeal and adjacent structures. (From Rakel RE: Saunders Manual of Medical Practice. Philadelphia, WB Saunders Co, 1996, p 157.)

4. Scalpel (no. 15 blade is ideal)
5. Retractors (Army-Navy retractors or large vein retractors)
6. Kelly clamp
7. Suture (2-0 or 3-0 silk, 4-0 Vicryl)
     Suture ligation of bleeders may be required. Suturing the
     tube in place also is important.
8. Assortment of cuffed tracheostomy tubes
     If these are not available, you may substitute no. 4 or 5
     small, flexible endotracheal (ET) tubes.

■ ANATOMY/APPROACH (Fig. 6–2)

The cricothyroid ligament lies between the cricoid and thyroid
cartilages in the neck. It is palpable in most patients with the
neck extended, as a recess located between the prominent thyroid
cartilage and the less prominent cricoid cartilage located about
1.5 cm inferior to the thyroid cartilage. Neck strap muscles lie
lateral to the cricothyroid ligament. Blood vessels, both arteries
and veins, lie just inferior to the ligament. Branches of the superior thyroid artery and the superficial thyroid veins are found
here.

■ ANESTHESIA

1. Local
     As described earlier, local anesthetic with epinephrine will
     decrease cutaneous bleeding and block the pain of skin inci-
     sion. However, pain from dissection in deeper planes is diffi-
     cult to control with a local anesthetic alone.
2. General or sedation
     It is rare that you will have the luxury of general anesthesia
     to perform a cricothyroidotomy. Generally, this procedure is
     performed in the environment of an emergency in which the
     airway has been lost. If a patient is awake and in distress,
     careful but rapid IV sedation can be provided to make the
     procedure easier for both the surgeon and the patient.
3. None
     In some emergency circumstances, cricothyroidotomy is per-
     formed on unconscious or comatose patients. In these cases,
     no anesthesia may be appropriate.

■ TECHNIQUE

1. Extend the patient's neck (avoid neck extension in patients
   with a cervical injury).
     Neck extension brings the cricothyroid membrane more
     superficially. Palpate the recess over the membrane.

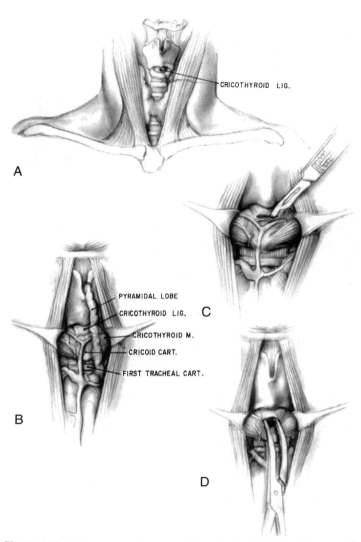

A

B

C

PYRAMIDAL LOBE

CRICOTHYROID LIG.

CRICOTHYROID M.

CRICOID CART.

FIRST TRACHEAL CART.

CRICOTHYROID LIG.

D

Figure 6–2 □ Anatomy and approach to cricothyroidotomy. (From Loré JM Jr: An Atlas of Head and Neck Surgery, 3rd ed. Philadelphia, WB Saunders Co, 1988, p 45.)

2. Inject local anesthetic with epinephrine if there is time; often, there is no time because the procedure is being done emergently in an unconscious patient.
3. Make a 3-cm horizontal or vertical skin incision centered over the cricothyroid membrane.

    Either incision is acceptable, yet each has advantages and disadvantages. A horizontal incision lessens the chance that the thyroid and cricoid cartilages will be damaged if the incision is carried too deeply. However, a vertical incision may be preferable in the neck of an obese patient in whom the cricothyroid membrane is not readily palpable.
4. Use a Kelly clamp to gently spread the subcutaneous tissue and to expose the cricothyroid membrane. Retractors may be needed to spread the neck strap muscles laterally to aid in exposure (see Fig. 6–2B).
5. Make a horizontal stab incision through the membrane, avoiding any visible blood vessels (see Fig. 6–2C).
6. The stab wound may be widened with the Kelly clamp as needed (see Fig. 6–2D).
7. Insert a tracheostomy tube or an ET.
8. Inflate the cuff of the tube, and secure the tube with sutures or tracheostomy ties.
9. Convert the cricothyroidotomy to a formal tracheostomy within 1 week.
10. Document the procedure.

■ COMPLICATIONS/PROBLEMS

1. Hemorrhage

    There are many vessels in the region of the cricothyroid membrane. Do your best to visualize and avoid these vessels.
2. Subglottic or glottic stenosis

    Cricothyroidotomy tubes left in place for more than 1 week have been shown to increase the risk of airway stenosis. Convert the cricothyroidotomy to a standard tracheostomy if a long-term airway below the larynx is needed.
3. Chondritis

    Inflammation and infection of the tracheal/cricoid cartilages or trachea can occur. It is best to keep patients with cricothyroidotomy on IV antibiotics directed against airway flora.

7

EMERGENCY TRACHEOSTOMY

This important procedure is more extensive than cricothyroidotomy (see Chapter 6) but more valuable for longer-term airway control and pulmonary toilet. In addition, tracheostomy poses less direct risk of vocal cord injury than cricothyroidotomy and provides a significantly larger airway. This procedure may be performed by the on-call team when the patient's airway is unstable and upper airway obstruction is present.

■ INDICATIONS

1. Obstruction of an airway in which oral or nasal intubation of the trachea cannot be performed
    Examples include laryngeal swelling, hematoma, vocal cord paralysis, and upper airway tumor.
2. Prolonged need for ventilatory support with an endotracheal tube (ET)
3. Subacute airway emergency
    If there is time to perform a tracheostomy semiemergently in the operating room, tracheostomy is preferable to cricothyroidotomy.

■ CONTRAINDICATIONS

1. Injudicious use
    This procedure should not be used in an on-call setting outside of emergent or semiemergent circumstances. Tracheostomy is associated with significant potential complications. To reduce these risks, an experienced surgical team should perform the tracheostomy in all except dire circumstances.
2. Coagulopathy
    Carefully consider the consequences of an invasive procedure such as tracheostomy. Bleeding into the trachea is a significant possibility in coagulopathic patients. The use of platelets, fresh frozen plasma, and other blood products may be needed to control procedural and postprocedural bleeding.
3. Known suprasternal location of the innominate artery

■ PRECAUTIONS

1. Know the regional anatomy to minimize the risk of injury to adjacent structures.
2. Use sterile technique if possible.

■ EQUIPMENT NEEDED

1. Adequate lighting
2. Suction
3. Local anesthesia if the patient is awake
     Consider the use of 1% lidocaine with 1:100,000 epinephrine to help minimize cutaneous bleeding.
4. A basic surgical set including
     a. Scalpel (both no. 11 and 15 blades are useful)
     b. Retractors (Army-Navy retractors or large vein retractors)
     c. Kelly clamps
     d. Needle drivers and pickups
5. Suture (2-0 or 3-0 silk, 4-0 Vicryl)
     Suture ligation of bleeders may be required. Suturing the tube in place also is important.
6. Assortment of cuffed tracheostomy tubes
     If these are not available, substitute no. 4 or 5 small, flexible tubes.

■ ANATOMY/APPROACH

The critical structures in the neck encountered during tracheostomy include the cricoid cartilage, thyroid gland, thyroid isthmus, strap muscles, and blood vessels. The important cross-sectional anatomy is shown in Figure 7–1.

■ ANESTHESIA

General; this procedure is too stimulating and uncomfortable to perform with local anesthesia or sedation.

■ TECHNIQUE

1. Hyperextend the head and neck, except in patients with cervical spine injuries.
2. About 1 to 2 cm below the cricoid cartilage, make a 4- to 5-cm incision either horizontally or vertically (Fig. 7–2).
     Horizontal incision is preferred. If making a vertical inci-

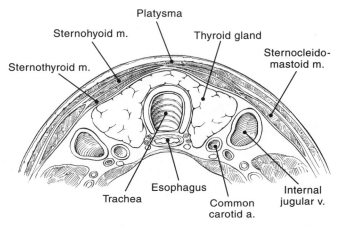

Platysma

Sternohyoid m.

Thyroid gland

Sternocleido-
mastoid m.

Sternothyroid m.

Esophagus

Internal
jugular v.

Trachea

Common
carotid a.

Figure 7–1 ◻ Cross-sectional anatomy of the neck. (From Rakel RE: Saunders Manual of Medical Practice. Philadelphia, WB Saunders Co, 1996, p 158.)

sion, care must be taken not to disturb the innominate artery, which may be above the sternal notch in 25% of patients (see Fig. 7–3A).

3. Carry the skin incision through the platysma muscle. Retract the skin flaps.
4. Make a vertical incision in the midline fascia between the strap muscles (Fig. 7–3B).
5. Look for the cricoid cartilage superiorly and the thyroid isthmus inferiorly (Fig. 7–3C).

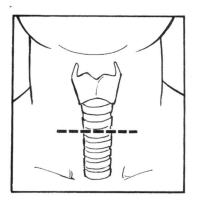

Figure 7–2 ◻ Preferred emergency tracheostomy skin incision. (From Rakel RE: Saunders Manual of Medical Practice. Philadelphia, WB Saunders Co, 1996, p 158.)

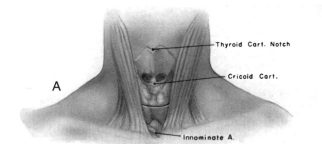

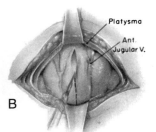

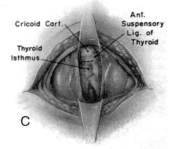

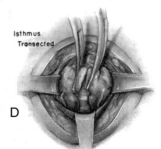

Figure 7–3 □ Surgical technique of tracheostomy. (From Loré JM Jr: An Atlas of Head and Neck Surgery, 3rd ed. Philadelphia, WB Saunders Co, 1988, pp 813, 815.)

Illustration continued on following page

6. Retract the thyroid isthmus superiorly to expose the second, third, and fourth tracheal rings.

   If the isthmus does not move with attempts at retraction, two curved clamps should be inserted across the isthmus, and the isthmus should be transected. Place suture ligatures around the cut isthmus ends before removing the clamps (Fig. 7–3D).

7. A no. 11 blade is carefully used to cut a window out of the trachea after first making a 5- to 8-mm horizontal incision directly above the tracheal ring of choice.

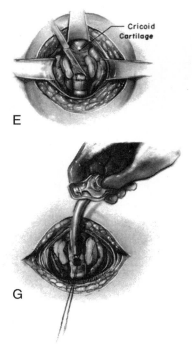

Cricoid
Cartilage

E   F

G

Figure 7–3 □ *Continued*

You may place the tracheostomy opening in the second, third, or fourth ring (Fig. 7–3*E*).

8. The incision then should be carried down across the ring and then back horizontally directly below the ring.

A small section of tracheal cartilage thus is removed. Removal of this small section reduces the risk of a piece of cartilage's being pushed into the tracheal lumen and reduces the risk of narrowing the tracheal airway from an inverted flap of trachea once the tracheostomy is removed (Fig. 7–3*F*).

9. Two heavy nylon or silk sutures should be placed in the trachea on both the right and left sides of the tracheal window.

Should the tracheostomy tube dislodge in the early postoperative period, these sutures serve as guides to help find the tracheal opening in the neck and facilitate replacement of a tracheostomy tube if necessary.

10. Quickly insert an appropriately sized tracheostomy tube with its obturator. Once the tube is inserted, remove the obturator (Fig. 7–3*G*).

If the patient is already orotracheally intubated, have an assistant slowly pull the endotracheal tube back until the tracheal lumen is visible. Then insert the tracheostomy tube.

11. Partially close the skin around the tracheostomy tube. Leave a small portion of the skin incision open along the tube to allow air to escape and to prevent tension emphysema.
12. Suture the tracheostomy tube to the skin with heavy nylon or silk sutures.
13. Secure the tracheostomy with tracheostomy ties.
14. Tape the ends of the lateral tracheal "safety" sutures to the skin along the trach tube.
15. Obtain a chest x-ray (CXR) to evaluate tube length and to rule out pneumothorax.
16. Document the procedure.

■ COMPLICATIONS/PROBLEMS

1. Injury to adjacent structures
   The esophagus, recurrent laryngeal nerves, and great vessels can be injured during the surgical procedure.
2. Pneumothorax
   This can be unilateral, bilateral, tension, or nontension.
3. Apnea or cardiac arrest
   This can follow from loss of airway and ventilation during the procedure. This is a significant risk in very obese patients, in whom loss of tracheal exposure and control can occur during surgery.
4. Tracheal perforation
5. Postoperative complications
   These include tracheoesophageal fistula, erosion of a great vessel, tracheal stenosis, infection, and aspiration.

If you note that the tracheostomy tube moves unduly with each heartbeat, suspect that the tracheostomy tube and trachea lie adjacent to a great vessel. In these cases, only very soft tracheostomy tubes should be used, and they should be pulled back to avoid lying adjacent to great vessels. If a rigid tracheostomy tube erodes through the trachea, great vessel erosion and exsanguinating hemorrhage can occur.

Tracheal stenosis is almost always due to tracheal cuff overinflation or overuse. The cuff on a tracheostomy tube should be used only when cuff function is needed to adequately ventilate a patient. Prolonged or incorrect use of the cuff leads to tracheal ischemia and eventually scarring and stenosis.

8

MASK VENTILATION: ORAL AND NASAL AIRWAYS

Mask Ventilation

Mask ventilation refers to assisted ventilation with a face mask. It is often the easiest means by which to ventilate a patient. The technique is relatively simple and quick and requires little invasive action. Two adjuncts to airway management—oral airways and nasopharyngeal airways—are also presented in this chapter. The techniques presented here can be used alone or in conjunction with endotracheal intubation.

■ INDICATIONS

1. Hypoventilation
2. Hypoxemia
3. Respiratory arrest

Mask ventilation is the first step in the initiation of ventilation and gas exchange for a patient with impending respiratory failure. Patients who are likely to require long-term respiratory support will likely require endotracheal intubation after masking. However, patients with short-term respiratory problems may be effectively treated with mask ventilation alone.

■ CONTRAINDICATION

1. Upper airway obstruction
   Obstruction would prevent mask-assisted ventilation from being effective.

■ PRECAUTIONS

1. Obesity
   Patients with obesity have a form of upper airway obstruction. The soft tissue mass of the cheeks and neck makes masking very difficult.

2. Airway-related infection

   Epiglottitis, bronchitis, and pneumonia cause airway irritability with cough, bronchospasm, and possible laryngospasm.

3. Facial trauma

   Facial fractures, such as mandibular or maxillary fractures, can create bleeding, swelling, and airway instability and obstruction.

4. Cervical spine injury

   Neck manipulation in the presence of neck trauma can damage the spinal cord.

5. Temporomandibular joint (TMJ) syndrome

   Patients with TMJ syndrome may have trismus, limited jaw opening, and even ankylosis of the jaw.

6. The use of an oral airway may induce gagging and vomiting, leading to aspiration. Use oral airways only when patients are anesthetized, when the oral airway is unlikely to stimulate the gag reflex.

■ EQUIPMENT NEEDED

1. Face mask

   Face masks are made of rubber or plastic and are available in a variety of sizes. For adults, use a small or medium size. For children, use a newborn, infant, or children's size.

2. Ambu bag

3. Oxygen

4. Oxygen saturation monitor

   It is important to assess oxygen saturation as a measurement of effective ventilation and gas exchange.

■ ANATOMY

The nasal airway is the predominant source of air inflow for most patients, and it acts to humidify the airstream (Fig. 8–1). The portion of the airway from the nose to the soft palate is known as the *nasopharynx*. In situations in which the nasal airway is obstructed or when greater air flow rates are needed, such as during exercise, mouth breathing occurs. Air moving into the mouth enters the oral airway, which extends from the anterior teeth to the base of the tongue. The portion of the airway extending from the posterior aspect of the nose to the cricoid cartilage is known as the *pharyngeal airway*.

Once air passes by either the oral or the nasal airway to the back of the throat, the air must pass between the posterior part of the tongue (base of tongue) and the posterior pharyngeal wall. It is common to have airway obstruction when the base of tongue

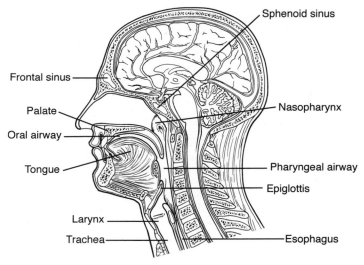

Figure 8–1 ▫ Anatomy of the oral and nasal airways.

falls posteriorly against the posterior pharyngeal wall. This creates airway obstruction and is commonly seen in patients who are lying supine.

Air passes from the pharynx into the larynx, where the vocal cords are located. Air must flow between the cords to pass into the trachea. Spasm of the cords and the muscles that control them causes laryngospasm.

■ TECHNIQUE

1. Hold the mask in one hand, using the thumb and index finger to push the mask down over the mouth. A tight fit is needed (Fig. 8–2).
2. The remaining three fingers should rest on the lower bony mandibular border, and an upward lifting force should be applied. These maneuvers simultaneously create mask seal and forward jaw thrust.
3. If adequate seal or jaw thrust cannot be obtained with one hand, use two hands to simultaneously create mask seal and forward jaw thrust. An assistant will be required to provide manual ventilation by squeezing the Ambu bag.
4. Watch for chest rise and fall, have an assistant listen for breath sounds, and watch the oxygen saturation carefully.

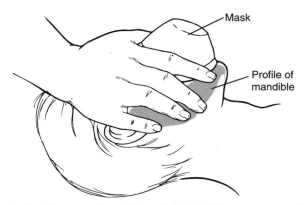

Mask

Profile of
mandible

Figure 8–2 □ Technique for mask ventilation. Hold the mask in one hand, using the thumb and index finger to push the mask down over the mouth. A tight fit is necessary.

■ COMPLICATIONS/PROBLEMS

1. Failure to adequately ventilate
   a. A poorly fitting mask can cause an air leak.
   b. Poor technique may be causing the problem.
      Be sure that the jaw is thrust forward, minimizing obstruction of the airway by the tongue.
   c. Rule out airway obstruction.
      This may be caused by the tongue, a foreign body, obesity, and other causes.
2. Insufflation of the stomach
   a. With mask ventilation with assisted breathing, it is possible to push air into the stomach. As the stomach becomes distended, it becomes harder to ventilate. In the unconscious patient, it is easy to pass a nasogastric tube to suction out this gastric air.

Oral Airway

The oral airway is a plastic, rigid device that is shaped somewhat like a question mark (Fig. 8–3). It has a hollow center, which allows air passage. When properly placed, the oral airway rides over the tongue and down along the tongue base. It holds the tongue base anteriorly and prevents obstruction by the tongue base against the posterior pharyngeal wall.

The oral airway is generally inserted with the tip up toward

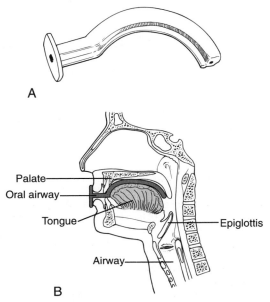

Figure 8–3 □ *A*, Oral airway; *B*, functional position of oral airway.

the palate and gently rotated 180° as it is passed posteriorly. The rigid oral airway should be used only on anesthetized or unconscious patients because it may provoke a gag reflex or may be followed by cough, vomiting, laryngospasm, and even bronchospasm.

Oral airways for adults are numbered 3, 4, and 5 and correspond to lengths of 80, 90, and 100 mm, respectively. Children's airways are numbered 0, 1, and 2 and correspond to lengths of 50, 60, and 70 mm, respectively.

Nasopharyngeal Airway

The nasopharyngeal airway is a soft, rubber tube that has many uses (Fig. 8–4). When properly placed, this airway passes through the nasopharynx down toward the laryngopharynx. These airways are well tolerated by patients and do not tend to stimulate significant gag reflexes.

The nasal airway is first lubricated with 2% lidocaine jelly. It is then passed through one side of the nose and into the nasal cavity. The airway is advanced to the full length. The tip of the

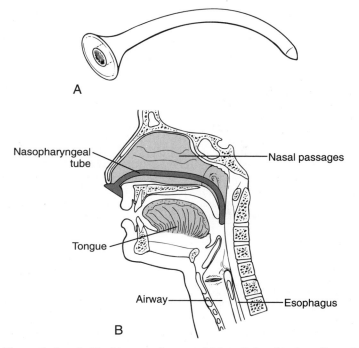

Figure 8–4 □ *A*, Flexible nasopharyngeal tube; *B*, functional position of tube.

airway should be inserted perpendicular to the face and not upward toward the cribriform plate. A good rule of thumb is that the length of the airway should be roughly the distance from the tip of the nose to the meatus of the ear.

Adult nasal airways are measured in French numbers, which relate to their outer diameter and circumference; popular sizes are 28, 30, 32, and 34. The airway has an outer flange that may be taped to the upper lip and cheek. When these airways are critical for maintenance of air flow, they may be sutured to the cutaneous portion of the nasal septum.

9

OROTRACHEAL INTUBATION

This chapter focuses on endotracheal intubation by the oral route. Orotracheal intubation is the most common way of obtaining emergent airway control when ventilation by mask is not appropriate or possible. This procedure requires an understanding of the pharyngeal and laryngeal anatomy, direct visualization of the vocal cords to ensure proper endotracheal tube placement, and an understanding of proper technique. If the operator is inexperienced in airway management and control, intubation efforts should be supervised by experienced personnel.

■ INDICATIONS

1. Airway protection
   An endotracheal tube, especially if the tube has a cuff, is a good way to protect the airway from aspiration.
2. Maintenance of patent airway
   In patients with airway instability and significant illness, the endotracheal tube maintains an open airway for the delivery of gases and for pulmonary toilet.
3. Opportunity to apply positive pressure ventilation
   With mask ventilation, it is difficult to apply positive pressure ventilation with significant pressures for long periods. Positive pressures delivered via mask frequently cause the stomach to fill with air, which makes continued ventilation difficult.
4. Pulmonary toilet
   Patients with poor pulmonary toilet and lung disease can benefit from simultaneous respiratory support and deep suctioning when an endotracheal tube is present.
5. Opportunity to maintain and control oxygenation by alteration of Fio_2, positive end-expiratory pressure (PEEP), and pressure support
   With an endotracheal tube in place, the ventilator can deliver oxygen in desired concentrations with end-expiratory pressure and pressure support. End-expiratory pressure helps keep small airways open. Pressure support makes the work of breathing with the ventilator easier for the ill patient. Ventilator settings can be gradually reduced as the condition of the patient improves.

■ CONTRAINDICATIONS

1. No clinical need for intubation

   If it is possible to manage the airway adequately without intubation, it is generally inappropriate to intubate. Intubation is associated with risks and potential complications. For example, inexperienced personnel can accidentally intubate the esophagus rather than the trachea. Unless detected rapidly, this error can lead to the death of the patient. Other problems, such as airway or dental trauma, can occur. Always ensure that the patient requires intubation before proceeding. The benefits should outweigh the risks!

2. Inaccessible oral cavity or extensive oral or laryngeal injury

   If a patient has his or her upper and lower jaws wired together, such as occurs after mandibular or maxillary fracture surgery, it is impossible to intubate orally. Other situations that may make oral intubation difficult or impossible include extensive oral trauma and bleeding, oral stenosis, severe temporomandibular joint disease, and scarring of the lips and mouth due to burns. In these difficult cases, nasal intubation is required. Enlist the help of an anesthesiologist to intubate nasally. Know that nasal intubation has several important contraindications, including coagulopathy, severe intranasal pathology, basilar skull fracture, and cerebrospinal fluid leak.

3. Cervical spine instability

   Neck extension in the presence of a cervical spine instability or trauma may lead to spinal cord injury. If a cervical spine injury is suspected, nasal intubation, fiberoptic-aided intubation, or a surgical airway may be appropriate.

■ PRECAUTIONS

1. Have a thorough understanding of the relevant airway anatomy. This will make intubation easier and safer for your patient.

2. Have oxygen, bag, mask, and suction at the bedside to maintain oxygenation and airway visibility during the procedure.

3. Have a laryngoscope with an assortment of blades at the bedside. Sometimes a straight blade is easier than a curved blade for visualization of the epiglottis and vocal cords. It is critical to have both types of blades available so you can choose whichever works best.

4. Have several different sizes of endotracheal tubes at the bedside. If too small a tube is used, an air leak may occur around the tube or the pulmonary toilet may be difficult. If too wide an endotracheal tube is used, trauma and ischemic injury to the laryngeal structures and trachea may occur.

5. If possible, have an assistant present to help you maintain positioning, apply downward pressure on the cricoid cartilage if necessary, or help you intubate (if he or she is more experienced than you).

■ EQUIPMENT NEEDED

1. Oxygen
2. Bag-valve-mask ventilation device
3. Suction
4. Oral suction tip (Yankauer tip) and soft, flexible suction catheter

    The oral suction tip is rigid and is used to suction the mouth and pharynx. The soft, flexible catheter is used for deeper suctioning.
5. Laryngoscope with both straight and curved blades

    The standard laryngoscope consists of a detachable blade with a removable bulb that connects to a battery-containing handle. The light becomes operational when the blade is fully extended. There are curved blades and straight blades. The curved blade, no. 3, is most frequently used for adult patients. Most operators start with the curved blade. In instances in which mouth opening is limited or visualization with the curved blade is difficult, the straight blade may be better for visualization.
6. Endotracheal tubes

    An assortment of different-sized tubes are needed. The majority of the endotracheal tubes that are used for adult intubation have a cuff balloon in the lower part of the tube. The cuff, when inflated appropriately, provides a seal so that air leak will be minimal during positive pressure ventilation. Cuffed endotracheal tubes also have a pilot balloon attached to the cuff. This device allows the operator a sense of how much tension is in the cuff when inflated with air. See Figure 9–1 for a diagram of a cuffed endotracheal tube and Table 9–1 for a guideline of what tube size is appropriate for a patient.
7. Flexible metal stylet

    The stylet is a flexible metal wire that can be inserted into the flexible endotracheal tube to increase its stiffness and to control its shape.
8. Syringes (two 10 ml) for cuff inflation
9. Magill forceps to direct the tube if needed

    These forceps are long and allow manipulation of the end of the endotracheal tube.
10. Water-soluble 2% lidocaine jelly to lubricate the endotracheal tube and stylet
11. Tape and skin adhesive to secure the endotracheal tube
12. Oxygen saturation monitor, if available

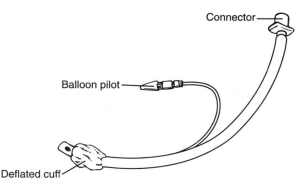

Figure 9–1 □ Cuffed endotracheal tube.

■ ANATOMY/APPROACH

The key anatomic landmarks for orotracheal intubation are the tongue base, vallecula, epiglottis, and vocal cords.

When looking down into the laryngopharynx from behind and above the patient, one must quickly orient to the anatomy (Fig. 9–2).

1. The tongue will be the most superior structure in the midline.
2. The tongue base will be just superior to the epiglottis.

Table 9–1 □ **ENDOTRACHEAL TUBE SIZE AND POSITION BASED ON PATIENT AGE**

Age	Tube Size (Internal diameter in cm)	Distance Inserted From Lips to Midtrachea (cm)
Premature infant	2.5	10
Full-term infant	3.0	11
1–6 mo	3.5	11
6–12 mo	4.0	12
2 y	4.5	13
4 y	5.0	14
6 y	5.5	15
8 y	6.0	16
10 y	6.5	17
12 y	7.0	18–22
14 y to adult	7.0	18–22
Female adult	7.0	20–24
Male adult	8.0	20–24

For nasal intubation, add 2 to 3 cm to the tube lengths provided in the table.

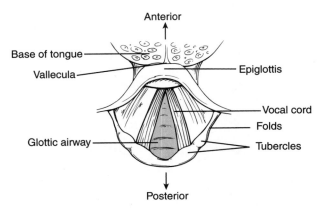

Anterior

Base of tongue——

Vallecula——

——Epiglottis

——Vocal cord

—— Folds

Glottic airway——

—— Tubercles

Posterior

Figure 9–2 □ Anatomy of the laryngopharynx.

3. The vallecula is the recess or space between the tongue base and epiglottis.
4. The vocal cords appear as two bands and are pale white.
5. The glottic opening is recognized by its triangular shape, and it is bound by the vocal cords.

 The endotracheal tube will be inserted through the glottic opening.

■ ANESTHESIA

 Endotracheal intubation is stimulating to the autonomic nervous system, and care must be taken to not stimulate aspiration. Consider the following guidelines:

1. If the patient is unconscious and orotracheal intubation is to be performed, generally no drugs are required.

 This situation is encountered frequently in emergent situations. For example, in many code situations and severe trauma cases, the patient is unconscious.
2. If the patient to be intubated is conscious, rapid-sequence intubation is generally used. In this technique, the risk of regurgitation and aspiration is reduced by the intravenous administration of a rapid-onset sedative/hypnotic agent and muscle relaxant with or without a narcotic analgesic agent.
 a. Thiopental (2 to 5 mg/kg IV)

 A lower initial dose (25 to 50 mg IV, repeated at 1- to 2-minute intervals) is recommended for ill patients or those with limited cardiovascular reserve.
 b. Succinylcholine (1.0 to 1.5 mg/kg IV)

This provides muscle relaxation. *Ensure that your patient is adequately sedated before administering this paralytic agent!*

c. Optional agents can be administered with thiopental, including the following:
   1. Fentanyl (25 to 50 μg IV) may be repeated as needed; morphine (2 to 5 mg) may be substituted for fentanyl. These agents increase sedation and offer analgesia.
   2. Lidocaine (1 mg/kg IV) can be used for increased intracranial pressure or reactive airway disease.
   3. Vecuronium (1 mg IV) can be used to prevent succinylcholine-induced fasciculations.

3. If the patient is awake, a topical anesthetic agent, a mild sedative, and an analgesic agent can be used to perform an awake intubation. This allows the patient to breathe spontaneously and leaves intact the airway protection reflexes.
   a. Benzocaine (20%) aerosol can be used to topically anesthetize the tongue and posterior pharynx.
   b. Midazolam (Versed) or thiopental can be used to provide sedation.
   c. Fentanyl or morphine is commonly used to add to sedation and analgesia.

■ TECHNIQUE

1. Quickly assess the airway. Remove dentures or foreign bodies from the mouth. Use the mask to ventilate the patient and to maximize oxygenation. If the patient is deeply sedated or unconscious, an oral airway can be inserted to help with the mask ventilation. Once the patient is well oxygenated, proceed with intubation as described. As always, use judgment in deciding how long to use the mask. If the airway is unstable and masking is difficult or impossible, proceed directly with intubation.
2. Align the oral, pharyngeal, and laryngeal axes by extending the head and flexing the neck (Fig. 9–3). A folded towel, foam material, or rubber "donut" placed under the occiput aids in the simultaneous flexion of the neck and maintenance of a padded surface for the head.
3. Have an assistant apply backward pressure to the anterolateral rim of the cricoid cartilage with the thumb and index finger (Fig. 9–4). In addition to occlusion of the esophagus, this maneuver often helps bring the larynx into view when the laryngoscope is used. This maneuver is maintained until proper placement of the endotracheal tube is clinically determined.
4. With the laryngoscope in the left hand, open the mouth with the fingers of the right hand and insert the laryngoscope blade into the right side of the mouth. Advance the blade midline to

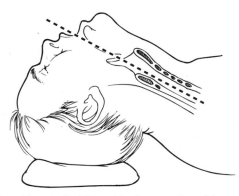

Figure 9–3 □ Alignment of the oral, pharyngeal, and laryngeal axes by extending the head and flexing the neck. (Redrawn from Rakel RE: Saunders Manual of Medical Practice. Philadelphia, WB Saunders Co, 1996.)

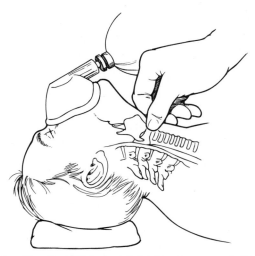

Figure 9–4 □ Have an assistant apply backward pressure to the anterolateral rim of the cricoid cartilage with the thumb and index finger. (Redrawn from Rakel RE: Saunders Manual of Medical Practice. Philadelphia, WB Saunders Co, 1996.)

the base of the tongue, sweeping the tongue leftward. If a curved blade is used, its tip should be inserted into the vallecula. Figure 9–5 shows visualization of the cords with the use of a curved blade. When a straight blade is used, its tip should be positioned below the epiglottis (Fig. 9–6). (These descriptions are for right-handed operators. If you are left-handed, use the opposite hands.)

5. Lift the handle of the laryngoscope upward and forward to expose the vocal cords. Avoid pressure on the lips and teeth. Also, watch to ensure that there is no entrapment of the tongue between the laryngoscope blade and teeth.

6. With the right hand, pass the lubricated endotracheal tube through the right corner of the mouth and advance the tip through the vocal cords under direct visualization. When the proximal end of the cuff is at the level of the cords, the stylet should be removed and the tube advanced into the trachea before the cuff is inflated. Ideally, the cuff should be inflated to about 15 mm Hg pressure. This usually corresponds to an easily compressible fullness in the balloon pilot. A manometer may be useful to gauge cuff pressure.

In men, the tube is generally inserted to about 23 cm at the lips to position the tube with the tip approximately 4 cm above the carina. For women, the distance is about 21 cm. For

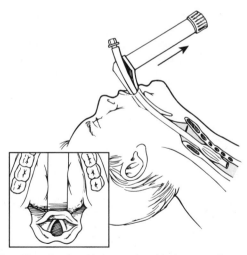

Figure 9–5 □ Visualization of the cords with the use of a curved blade. (Redrawn from Rakel RE: Saunders Manual of Medical Practice. Philadelphia, WB Saunders Co, 1996.)

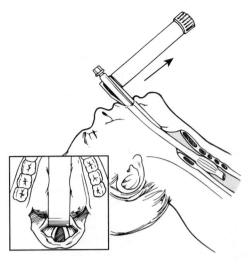

Figure 9–6 □ Positioning of a straight blade with its tip below the epiglottis. (Redrawn from Rakel RE: Saunders Manual of Medical Practice. Philadelphia, WB Saunders Co, 1996.)

children, the distance in centimeters at the lips can be estimated with the formula [12 + (age/2)].

7. Assess the patient for proper tube placement. Look for symmetric chest expansion, and listen for equal breath sounds over bilateral lung fields. Diminished breath sounds on the left may indicate right mainstem intubation. Also auscultate over the epigastric area as you are ventilating through the endotracheal tube. Gurgling sounds with ventilation may indicate esophageal intubation. If this is suspected, immediately remove the tube, ventilate with the mask, and reintubate. Rising oxygen saturation and the return of sufficient carbon dioxide during exhalation (with capnography) are useful in confirming tracheal intubation.

8. Secure the tube with tape over the upper lip and cheek. If a mustache or beard is present, the tube may be tied in position and secured around the head.

9. Always confirm the proper depth of tube placement with a chest x-ray (CXR).

■ COMPLICATIONS/PROBLEMS

1. Difficulty in visualizing vocal cords
   This is often due to poor head positioning, lack of downward cricoid cartilage pressure, or improper laryngoscope

Table 9–2 □ **PATIENTS AT HIGH RISK FOR ASPIRATION**

Full stomach (<6 hr after eating)
Obesity
Pregnancy
Trauma
Intestinal obstruction
Gastric paresis
Esophageal disease
Inability to recall last oral intake

blade selection. Ensure that the patient's head is extended, the mouth and oropharynx are properly suctioned, and the laryngoscope blade is either in the depth of the vallecula (curved blade) or below the epiglottis (straight blade).

2. Endotracheal tube in esophagus

   If you suspect that the endotracheal tube is in the esophagus, pull out the tube and begin mask ventilation. Once the patient is adequately oxygenated, try to intubate the trachea. Failure to recognize esophageal intubation may lead to death.

3. Mainstem bronchus intubation

   Listen carefully to breath sounds after intubating. Always look for evidence of a mainstem intubation; most mainstem intubations will be on the right side because of the bronchial anatomy. Always check a CXR. Remember that for adults, the tip of the tube should be about 4 cm above the carina. It may be necessary to pull back on the endotracheal tube if the tube tip is too close to the carina. Failure to recognize a mainstem intubation may lead to severe atelectasis, hypoxemia, and other complications.

4. Aspiration

   Some patients are at risk of aspiration of the gastric contents during intubation. Mortality rates due to aspiration after intubation may be as high as 5%. Table 9–2 lists the patients at a high risk for aspiration. Perform intubation on these patients only in emergent situations. Table 9–3 provides a list of tech-

Table 9–3 □ **TECHNIQUES AND AGENTS TO REDUCE ASPIRATION RISK AND ITS CONSEQUENCES**

Nothing by mouth for >6 hr: Reduces gastric content
Antacid administration: Reduces gastric acidity
Histamine H_2–blocking agents: Reduces gastric acidity
Metoclopramide (Reglan): Enhances gastric emptying
Rapid-sequence induction: Reduces stimulation of gag reflexes
Head-up positioning: Provides gravitational advantage

niques and agents that reduce aspiration risk or ameliorate its consequences.

5. Damage to the teeth

The laryngoscope is a hard device, and significant upward traction on the laryngoscope is required to view the larynx in many cases. However, when using the laryngoscope, always be careful to not apply pressure on the teeth, gums, or lips. This will help avoid a dental injury.

INTRAVASCULAR ACCESS

□ □ □

10

SELDINGER TECHNIQUE

This is a routine technique for placing intravascular lines. It is based on cannulating the vessel with a needle and passing a wire through the needle into the vessel. Once the wire is is placed in the vessel, the passageway through the tissues may be suitably widened by means of a rigid dilator. A large-bore catheter then may be placed over the wire.

■ INDICATIONS

This technique may be used any time an intravascular line is required. This technique also is used to place catheters into large body cavities such as during drainage of an abscess or placement of a tracheostomy tube. The technique described is for placement of an intravascular line.

■ CONTRAINDICATIONS

Any percutaneous approach to intravascular access is contraindicated in settings of skin lesions or infection overlying the site of insertion. Known thrombosis of the desired vessel is also a contraindication.

■ PRECAUTIONS

Refer also to the precautions for each specific approach.

1. Coagulopathy
   Abnormalities in platelet count or function or in clotting factor concentrations should be corrected before insertion of the line.
2. Ongoing systemic infection
   A peripheral site may be advisable until the source of infection is identified and suitable treatment has been begun. This may not always be possible.
3. Any time a guide wire is used, there is a risk of vessel perforation.

■ EQUIPMENT NEEDED

There are specific kits available for many approaches. Refer to the instructions supplied with these kits for complete information.

1. Skin preparation supplies (iodine, chlorhexidine, or alcohol)
2. Local anesthetic (1% or 2% lidocaine, 25-gauge needle, 3-ml syringe)
3. Sterile gloves
4. Sterile towels or drapes
5. Supplies for Seldinger technique (or specific intravascular access kit)
   a. Needle (16 to 18 gauge)
   b. 10-ml syringe
   c. Guide wire
   d. Scalpel
   e. Dilator
   f. Catheter
6. If the Seldinger technique is not used, a catheter-over-needle system may be used.
7. Heparinized saline for flushing the catheter
8. Suture for securing the catheter
9. Equipment for continuous monitoring of arterial or venous pressure, if desired
10. Sterile dressing supplies

■ ANATOMY/APPROACH

See the technique for each individual intravascular access approach.

■ ANESTHESIA

Local

■ TECHNIQUE (STERILE SELDINGER) (Fig. 10–1)

1. **Prepare the patient.**
   a. Explain the procedure.
   b. Explain the risks and alternatives. Obtain consent if necessary.
   c. Answer any questions.
2. **Position the patient.**
   a. Confirm that all the equipment is available.
   b. Prepare the equipment for use. Remove any unnecessary

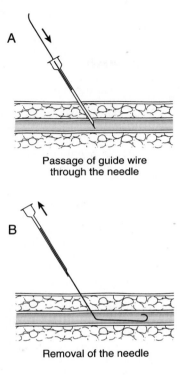

A

Passage of guide wire
through the needle

B

Removal of the needle

C

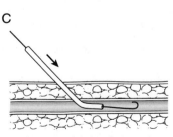

Passage of the catheter over
the guide wire

Figure 10–1 □ Seldinger technique for placing intravascular lines.

tags or covers, crack the seals of syringes, and remove the cap from the distal port of the line to be placed.
c. Position the patient as per each individual technique.

3. **Prepare the skin.**
   a. Use sterile technique.
   b. Prepare and drape the skin.
   c. Infiltrate the entry site with 1% to 2% lidocaine.
   d. Confirm that adequate anesthesia has been achieved.
      Pinch the skin over where the local anesthetic has been injected to test for a pain response.

4. **Place the 10-ml syringe on the needle.**
   Identify appropriate anatomic landmarks with the index finger of your nondominant hand.

5. **Insert the needle into the vessel.**
   Aspirate during insertion **and** during withdrawal, as often the vessel is encountered on the way out.

6. **When blood flows freely into the syringe, remove the syringe from the needle.**
   Immediately place your finger over the hub to stop the outflow of blood and to avoid the inflow of air.

7. **Gently place the guide wire through the needle** (see Fig. 10–1*A*)
   Ensure that the wire passes without resistance. It should feel like passing through warm butter. If you examine the guide wire before starting the procedure, you will note that as the wire bumps against a wall it will bend toward the curve of the J (Fig. 10–2). This may be exploited when a difficult placement is anticipated. Insert the wire in the orientation such that it will tend to bend toward the direction that you desire.
   If the wire does not pass easily, **do not force it.** Remove the needle and the guide wire together, and reposition the needle before reinsertion of the wire.
   If the patient is monitored, watch for ventricular dysrhythmias. This is an indication that the wire is too deep and should be pulled back until the dysrhythmias stop.

8. **Remove the needle over the wire** (see Fig. 10–1*B*)

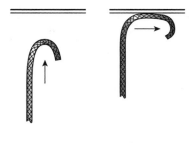

Figure 10–2 □ Typical bending pattern of J-wires. (From Adams GA, Bresnick SD: On Call Surgery. Philadelphia, WB Saunders Co, 1997, p 235.)

Always keep one hand on the wire to maintain its position in the vessel and to avoid the calamity of losing the wire completely in the vessel. (Don't let your patient's x-ray be the subject at the next interventional radiology grand rounds.)

9. **Nick the skin at the entry site with a scalpel.**
   Make the skin defect just large enough to allow passage of the catheter.

10. **Place the dilator over the wire, dilate the entry path, and then remove.**
    Often, a twisting motion is required. Do this close to the skin insertion site. Anticipate increased bleeding at the skin site on removal of the dilator. This is easily controlled with gentle pressure. Be careful to maintain the wire position.

11. **Place the catheter over the wire into the vessel** (see Fig. 10–1C)
    a. Maintain control of the wire.
    b. Remember to have removed the appropriate (distal) cap on multilumen catheters so that the wire passes through easily.
    c. It is advisable to have flushed the lumens of the catheter with heparinized saline before placement.
    d. Introducer sheaths for Swan-Ganz catheters should be introduced slowly because they become warm and more compliant as they enter the body. The introducers are very large, and rapid movements can damage a wider area.
    e. If the catheter slides easily into the lumen of the vessel, remove the wire. Hold your finger over the hub of the catheter until it is flushed and tightly capped.
    f. Confirm that each cap is in place and is tightly fastened.

12. **Confirm placement by aspirating blood from each port.**
    Flush each port with heparinized saline. Some lines require placement confirmation by x-ray before use.

13. **Secure the catheter at the skin level with suture.**

14. **Sterilely dress the site.**

15. **Document the procedure.**

■ COMPLICATIONS/PROBLEMS

See the technique for each individual intravascular access approach.

■ MANAGEMENT/FOLLOW-UP/REMOVAL

See the technique for each individual intravascular access approach.

11

CHANGING A LINE OVER A WIRE

This is a technique for replacing intravascular lines. It is a modification of the Seldinger technique, by which a guide wire is placed through the lumen of an existing line, and may be used only if the existing line and line site are free of infection.

■ INDICATIONS

This technique may be used any time an intravascular line change is required. The timing of a line change is a highly variable issue; check with the primary care team as to the interval and style of line change that are desirable.

■ CONTRAINDICATIONS

Any percutaneous approach to intravascular access is contraindicated in settings of skin lesions or infection overlying the site of insertion.

■ PRECAUTIONS

Refer to the precautions for each specific approach.

1. Coagulopathy
   Abnormalities in platelet count or function or in clotting factor concentrations should be corrected before insertion of the line.
2. Ongoing systemic infection
   A peripheral site may be advisable until the source of infection is identified and suitable treatment has been begun. This may not always be possible.
3. Any time a guide wire is used, there is a risk of vessel perforation.

■ EQUIPMENT NEEDED

Often, the same type of kit used to place the original line is needed. Refer to the instructions supplied with these kits for complete information.

1. Skin preparation supplies (iodine, chlorhexidine, or alcohol)
2. Local anesthetic (1% or 2% lidocaine, 25-gauge needle, 3-ml syringe)
3. Sterile gloves
4. Sterile towels or drapes
5. Supplies for Seldinger technique (or specific intravascular access kit)
    a. Needle (16 to 18 gauge)
    b. 10-ml syringe
    c. Guide wire
    d. Scalpel
    e. Dilator
    f. Catheter
       (Note that if there is difficulty with the line change, a complete kit is useful to have at the ready in order to start a completely new line.)
6. Heparinized saline for flushing the catheter
7. Suture for securing the catheter
8. Equipment for continuous monitoring of arterial or venous pressure, if desired
9. Sterile dressing supplies

■ ANATOMY/APPROACH

See the technique for each individual intravascular access approach.

■ ANESTHESIA

Local

■ TECHNIQUE (STERILE SELDINGER) (Fig. 11–1)

1. **Prepare the patient.**
    a. Explain the procedure.
    b. Explain the risks and alternatives. Obtain consent if necessary.
    c. Answer any questions.
2. **Position the patient.**
    a. Confirm that all the equipment is available.
    b. Prepare the equipment for use. Remove any unnecessary tags or covers, crack the seals of syringes, and remove the cap from the distal port of the line to be placed.

A

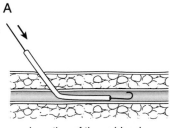

Insertion of the guide wire
through the old catheter

B

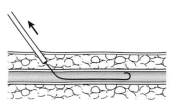

Removal of the old catheter

C

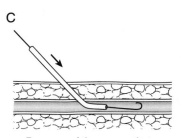

Passage of the new catheter
over the guide wire

Figure 11–1 □ Modification of
Seldinger technique for changing
a line over a wire.

   c. Position the patient as per each individual technique, generally supine.

3. Prepare the skin.

   a. Use sterile technique.

   b. Prepare and drape the skin.

   c. Infiltrate the suture sites with 1% to 2% lidocaine.

   d. Confirm that adequate anesthesia has been achieved.

      The local anesthetic is used to place the sutures at the end of the line placement and is not necessary at the entry site for the changing of the line. It is possible to wait until sutures are required before infiltrating the skin.

   e. It is important to prep the catheter very well.

      Pay special attention to the distal port through which the wire will pass.

4. Remove the cap from the distal port and place a finger over the end.

5. Gently place the guide wire through the distal port (see Fig. 11–1*A*).

      Ensure that the wire passes without resistance. It should feel like it is passing through warm butter. If the wire does not pass easily, **do not force it.**

6. Remove the catheter over the wire (see Fig. 11–1*B*).

      Always keep one hand on the wire to maintain its position in the vessel. If so desired, the tip of the catheter may be cut off with sterile scissors and sent for culture. Hold pressure at the skin site to avoid excessive bleeding.

7. Place the new catheter over the wire into the wound (see Fig. 11–1*C*).

   a. Maintain control of the wire.

   b. Remember to have removed the appropriate cap on multilumen catheters so that the wire passes through easily.

   c. It is advisable to have flushed the lumens of the catheter with heparinized saline before placement.

   d. Introducer sheaths for Swan-Ganz catheters should be introduced slowly because they become warm and more compliant as they enter the body. The introducers are very large, and rapid movements can damage a wider area.

   e. If the catheter slides easily into the lumen of the vessel, remove the wire. Hold your finger over the hub of the catheter until it is flushed and tightly capped.

   f. Confirm that each cap is in place and is tightly fastened.

8. Confirm placement by aspirating blood from each port.

      Flush each port with heparinized saline. Some lines require placement confirmation by x-ray before use.

9. Secure the catheter at the skin level with suture.

10. Sterilely dress the site.

11. Document the procedure.

■ COMPLICATIONS/PROBLEMS

See the technique for each individual intravascular access approach.

■ MANAGEMENT/FOLLOW-UP/REMOVAL

See the technique for each individual intravascular access approach.

12

CUTDOWN APPROACH

■ INDICATIONS

The cutdown approach for intravascular cannulation may be used for venous or arterial lines. This approach is reserved for situations in which percutaneous sites have been exhausted or when speed is of the essence.

■ CONTRAINDICATIONS

Any approach to intravascular access is contraindicated in settings of skin lesions or infection overlying the site of insertion.

■ PRECAUTIONS

1. Coagulopathy
   Abnormalities in platelet count or function or in clotting factor concentrations should be corrected before insertion of the line.
2. Ongoing systemic infection
   A peripheral site may be advisable until the source of infection is identified and suitable treatment has been begun. This may not always be possible.
3. Dislodgment of these lines
   This can result in rapid exsanguination.

■ EQUIPMENT NEEDED

Often, specific cutdown trays are available. The equipment listed below is generally on them.

1. Skin preparation supplies (iodine, chlorhexidine, or alcohol)
2. Local anesthetic (1% or 2% lidocaine, 25-gauge needle, 3-ml syringe)
3. Sterile gloves
4. Sterile towels or drapes
5. Catheter (18- to 22-gauge angiocatheter)
6. Cutdown kit
   a. 3-0 or 4-0 silk sutures
   b. No. 10 and 11 blade scalpels

    c. Scalpel holder
    d. Curved hemostats (2)
    e. Gauze sponges
    f. Scissors
    g. Needle driver
    h. Skin retractors
    i. Syringes
  7. Heparinized saline in a pressurized delivery system (for arterial lines)
  8. Blood gas syringe if needed for arterial blood sampling
  9. Additional 5-ml syringe with heparinized saline
10. Suture for securing the catheter
11. Equipment for continuous monitoring of arterial pressure
12. Sterile dressing supplies

■ ANATOMY/APPROACH

Saphenous Venous Line

The saphenous vein is found 1 cm anterior and 1 cm superior to the medial malleolus on the ankle (Fig. 12–1).

Radial Arterial Line

The pulse of the radial artery is easily palpable on the volar surface of the wrist at the radial head (Fig. 12–2).

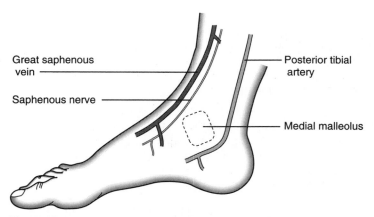

Great saphenous vein

Saphenous nerve

Posterior tibial artery

Medial malleolus

Figure 12–1 □ Medial view of ankle region and structures of major importance. (From Adams GA, Bresnick SD: On Call Surgery. Philadelphia, WB Saunders Co, 1997, p 259.)

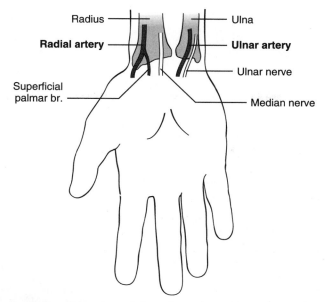

Figure 12–2 □ Volar view of the wrist region and structures of major importance.

■ ANESTHESIA

Local

■ TECHNIQUE (STERILE) (Fig. 12–3)

1. **Prepare the patient.**
   a. Explain the procedure.
   b. Explain the risks and alternatives. Obtain consent if necessary.
   c. Answer any questions.
2. **Position the patient.**
   a. Position the patient supine.
   b. Confirm that all the equipment is available.
3. **Prepare the skin.**
   a. Use sterile technique.
   b. Prepare and drape the skin.
   c. Infiltrate the entry site with 1% to 2% lidocaine. Also infiltrate over the line of the incision and at the sites of anchoring sutures.

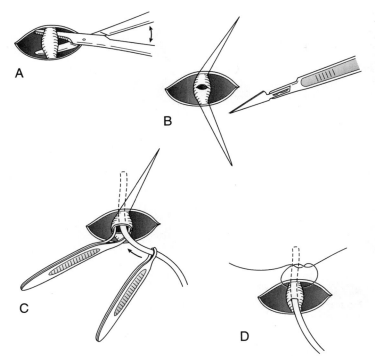

A. Isolation of vessel
B. Venotomy or arteriotomy
C. Placement of catheter
D. Securing catheter
E. Closure of incision

Figure 12–3 □ Technique for cutdown approach.

4. **Locate the vessel by palpation.**
5. **Make a skin incision over the vessel.**
   a. Make a transverse incision 1 to 1.5 cm in length.
   b. The vessel should be visible beneath the fascia.
6. **Bluntly dissect down to the vessel** (see Fig. 12–3A).
   a. Use hemostats to bluntly dissect alongside the vessel.
   b. Gently spread along the vessel course.

Spreading in a direction perpendicular to the course of the vessel is less likely to damage small branches.

7. **Gain proximal and distal control of the vessel** (see Fig. 12–3B).
   a. When the vessel is cleaned of investing tissue, gently spread underneath along the course of the vessel.
   b. Pass a silk suture under the vessel and pull proximally for occlusion and traction. Repeat with a second silk suture for distal control.

8. **Ligate the distal end of the vessel, if desired.**
   a. The distal control suture may be used.
   b. Ligation is **not** necessary and should be **avoided** in arterial line placements.

9. **Nick the vessel.**
   a. Enter as distal as possible along the exposed vessel.
   b. Fine scissors or a No. 11 blade may be used.
   c. The vessel lumen may be widened with a specific vessel dilator or with the tips of a fine hemostat.
   c. Alternatively, an angiocatheter may be used to directly enter the vessel before nicking it.

10. **Place the catheter into the vessel** (see Fig. 12–3C).
   This may be done directly through the nick in the vessel, or it may be tunneled through the skin through a separate distal stab incision.

11. **Secure the catheter in place** (see Fig. 12–3D).
   Tie down the proximal stay suture over the vessel and catheter. Take care not to tie this too tight, or the suture will cut through.

12. **Confirm adequate placement by aspiration.**

13. **Close the skin with 4-0 sutures** (see Fig. 12–3E).

14. **Apply a sterile dressing.**

15. **Document the procedure.**

■ COMPLICATIONS/PROBLEMS OF CUTDOWN SITES

1. Nonplacement of the line
2. Entry site infection
   The line must be removed and a new site used, if necessary.
3. Vessel thrombosis
   Transient occlusion is common, occurring in about 10% of arterial line placements. It is treated with removal of the line.
4. Suppurative thrombophlebitis
   This may require surgical drainage and IV antibiotics.
5. Distal ischemia
   Remove the line.
6. Bleeding from the placement site

Be sure to check the connections.

Under arterial pressures, a poor coupling of lines can result in rapid exsanguination.

If the bleeding is venous, tie down the distal side of the vessel if this has not already been done. Occasionally, a stitch at the entry site will suffice.

7. Nonfunction

■ REMOVAL OF LINES PLACED BY CUTDOWN

1. Have ready a scissors or blade, gauze, and tape.
2. Always wear gloves when there is a potential for exposure to blood or other body fluids.
3. Remove sutures.
4. Remove the catheter.
5. Apply firm pressure at the entry site.

   If the site was arterial, hold pressure for 10 minutes (by the clock) and longer if the lumen was large or if the patient is anticoagulated.
6. Confirm that bleeding has stopped.
7. Place a pressure dressing.
8. Check the site and confirm adequate blood flow to the extremity the next day.

ARTERIAL LINES

□ □ □

13

PERIPHERAL ARTERIAL LINE WITH ANGIOCATHETER

The most straightforward approach involves the placement of a simple angiocatheter in the wrist. There are arterial line kits available that use the Seldinger (guide wire) technique that also are acceptable. The dorsalis pedis artery also may be used with this technique.

■ INDICATIONS

Indications are hemodynamic monitoring, arterial blood sampling, and frequent blood draw requirements in the nonambulatory patient. Placement of arterial lines is generally done in an ICU setting, where the patient is under close observation.

■ CONTRAINDICATIONS

Any percutaneous approach to intravascular access is contraindicated in settings of skin lesions or infection overlying the site of insertion.

■ PRECAUTIONS

1. Coagulopathy
   Abnormalities in platelet count or function or in clotting factor concentrations should be corrected before insertion of the line.
2. Ongoing systemic infection
3. Dislodgment of these lines
   This can result in rapid exsanguination.

■ EQUIPMENT NEEDED

1. Skin preparation supplies (iodine, chlorhexidine, or alcohol)
2. Local anesthetic (1% or 2% lidocaine, 25-gauge needle, 3-ml syringe)
3. Angiocatheter (20 or 22 gauge, 2 inches in length) or specific arterial line kit
4. Sterile gloves
5. Sterile towel or drapes
6. Heparinized saline in a pressurized delivery system
7. Blood gas syringe if needed for arterial blood sampling
8. Additional 5-ml syringe with heparinized saline
9. Suture for securing the catheter
10. Arm board with a small terry cloth roll to help secure line and prevent kinking
11. Equipment for continuous monitoring of arterial pressure
12. Sterile dressing supplies

■ ANATOMY/APPROACH

Select the site.

Radial Artery

The pulse of the radial artery is easily palpable on the volar surface of the wrist at the radial head (Fig. 13–1).

1. Perform an Allen test to confirm the collateral circulation in the hand.

    The Allen test is performed by compression of both the radial and ulnar arteries until the palm blanches; then, release the ulnar artery and confirm reperfusion of the palm. A delay of more than 5 seconds is considered abnormal, and another site should be chosen.
2. Whenever possible, choose the nondominant hand.

Dorsalis Pedis Artery

The dorsalis pedis artery is located on the dorsum of the foot at the midline, just below the ankle (Fig. 13–2).

■ ANESTHESIA

Local

■ TECHNIQUE (STERILE)

1. **Prepare the patient.**
    a. Explain the procedure.

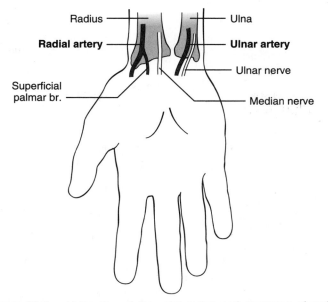

Figure 13–1 □ Volar view of the wrist region and structures of major importance.

   b. Explain the risks and alternatives. Obtain consent if necessary.

   c. Answer any questions.

2. Position the patient.

   a. The patient may be seated or supine. The selected wrist should be immobilized on an arm board with a roll under the wrist in slight dorsiflexion (Fig. 13–3).

   b. Get a chair for yourself.

   c. Raise the bed to a comfortable height.

   d. Confirm that all the equipment is available.

3. Prepare the skin.

   a. Use sterile technique.

   b. Prepare and drape the skin.

   c. Infiltrate the entry site with 1% to 2% lidocaine. Also infiltrate over the sites of anchoring sutures.

   d. Confirm that adequate anesthesia has been achieved.

4. Insert the catheter.

   a. After confirming that adequate anesthesia has been achieved, locate the pulse with the index finger of your nondominant hand.

   b. An optional step is to nick the skin over the entry site with

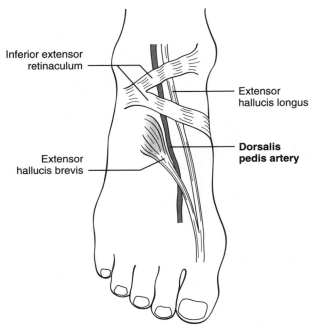

Figure 13–2 □ Dorsal view of the foot and structures of major importance.

    a scalpel in order not to damage the catheter as it enters the skin.

    c. Insert the angiocatheter at a 30° to 45° angle to the artery.

    d. When bright red blood pumps freely into the catheter, continue to advance the catheter slowly until the flow just stops.

    e. Back off slightly until the blood pumps again, and advance the catheter over the needle into the vessel.

5. If blood does not immediately flow into the needle

    a. Pull out, reconfirm the landmarks, reposition, and try again.

    b. Occasionally, the needle needs to be flushed of clogging tissue before reinsertion. Use a syringe of heparinized saline.

    c. If the catheter cannot be placed in three attempts, try another site.

6. When the catheter is successfully placed

    a. Secure the catheter to the skin with suture.
        Some angiocatheters have wings for this purpose.

    b. Obtain arterial blood samples as needed.

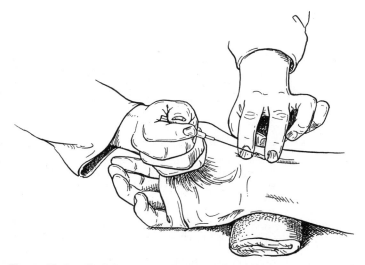

Figure 13–3 □ Radial artery cannulation. (From Dunmire SM, Paris PM: Atlas of Emergency Procedures. Philadelphia, WB Saunders Co, 1995, p 199.)

   c. Attach to manometer for continuous monitoring.
   d. Apply a sterile dressing.
7. Document the procedure.
8. General considerations
   a. Reassess daily the need for the arterial line.
   b. Confirm daily adequate blood flow to the hand and fingers.
   c. If fever occurs, remember to draw blood for cultures from this site as well as from other indwelling sites.
   d. If the site remains clean, the catheter may be changed over a wire as needed.

■ COMPLICATIONS/PROBLEMS

1. Nonplacement of the line
2. Entry site infection
    The line must be removed and a new site used, if necessary.
3. Vessel thrombosis
    Transient occlusion is common, occurring in about 10% of placements. It is treated with removal of the line.
4. Suppurative thrombophlebitis
    This may require surgical drainage and IV antibiotics.

5. Distal ischemia
   Remove the line. Confirm distal pulses.
6. Bleeding from the placement site
   Be sure to check the connections. Under arterial pressures, a poor coupling of lines can result in rapid exsanguination. Occasionally, a stitch at the entry site will suffice.
7. Nonfunction

■ REMOVAL OF ARTERIAL LINES

1. Have a scissors or blade, gauze, and tape ready.
2. Always wear gloves when there is a potential for exposure to blood or other body fluids.
3. Remove sutures.
4. Remove the catheter.
5. Apply firm pressure at the entry site for 10 minutes (by the clock) and longer if the lumen was large or if the patient was anticoagulated.
6. After 10 minutes, confirm that bleeding has stopped.
7. Place a pressure dressing.
8. Check the site and confirm adequate blood flow to the extremity the next day.

14

FEMORAL ARTERIAL LINE BY SELDINGER TECHNIQUE

This technique is used in supine patients in whom the radial or dorsal pedal approach has failed or is not possible.

■ INDICATIONS

Indications are hemodynamic monitoring, arterial blood sampling, and frequent blood draw requirements in the nonambulatory patient. Placement of arterial lines is generally done in an ICU setting, where the patient is under close observation.

■ CONTRAINDICATIONS

Any percutaneous approach to intravascular access is contraindicated in settings of skin lesions or infection overlying the site of insertion.

■ PRECAUTIONS

1. Coagulopathy
    Abnormalities in platelet count or function or in clotting factor concentrations should be corrected before insertion of the line.
2. Ongoing systemic infection
3. Dislodgment of these lines
    This can result in rapid exsanguination.

■ EQUIPMENT NEEDED

1. Skin preparation supplies (iodine, chlorhexidine, or alcohol)
2. Local anesthetic (1% or 2% lidocaine, 25-gauge needle, 3-ml syringe)
3. Sterile gloves
4. Sterile towels or drapes
5. Supplies for Seldinger technique (or specific arterial line kit)
    a. Needle (16 to 18 gauge)
    b. 10-ml syringe

    c. Guide wire
    d. Scalpel
    e. Dilator
    f. Catheter
6. If the Seldinger technique is not used, a catheter-over-needle system may be used.
7. Heparinized saline in a pressurized delivery system
8. Blood gas syringe if needed for arterial blood sampling
9. Additional 5-ml syringe with heparinized saline
10. Suture for securing the catheter
11. Equipment for continuous monitoring of arterial pressure
12. Sterile dressing supplies

■ ANATOMY/APPROACH

Select the site.

1. Recall the orientation of the vessels in the groin.
    The artery is found halfway between the anterior iliac spine and the symphysis pubis (Fig. 14–1).
2. Palpate the groin to assess for adequate pulse.
3. Document the presence of distal pulses in the desired extremity.

■ ANESTHESIA

Local

■ TECHNIQUE (STERILE SELDINGER)

1. **Prepare the patient.**
    a. Explain the procedure.

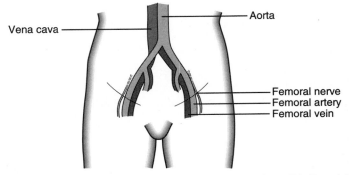

Figure 14–1 □ Anatomy of groin vasculature. (From Adams GA, Bresnick SD: On Call Surgery. Philadelphia, WB Saunders Co, 1997, p 239.)

b. Explain the risks and alternatives. Obtain consent if necessary.

c. Answer any questions.

2. Position the patient.

a. The patient must be supine.

b. Raise the bed to a comfortable height.

c. Confirm that all the equipment is available.

3. Prepare the skin.

a. Use sterile technique.

b. Prepare and drape the skin. Shaving may be necessary.

c. Infiltrate the entry site with 1% to 2% lidocaine. Also infiltrate the sites of anchoring sutures.

d. Confirm that adequate anesthesia has been achieved.

4. Insert the catheter.

a. After confirming that adequate anesthesia has been achieved, locate the pulse with the index finger of your nondominant hand.

b. An optional step is to nick the skin over the entry site with a sterile scalpel in order not to damage the catheter as it enters the skin.

c. Place the 10-ml syringe on the needle and locate the pulse with the index finger of your nondominant hand.

d. Insert the needle at a 45° angle to the artery (about 3 to 4 cm). Aspirate during insertion **and** withdrawal because often the vessel is encountered on the way out.

e. When bright red blood pumps freely into the syringe, remove the syringe and immediately place your finger over the hub of the needle.

f. Place the guide wire through the needle. Make sure that the wire passes **without resistance.** Remove the needle over the wire. Be sure to control the wire.

g. Nick the skin at the entry site with a scalpel.

h. Place the dilator over the wire and then remove. Watch for increased bleeding at the skin site. This is easily controlled with gentle pressure.

i. Place the catheter over the wire into the wound.

j. Remove the wire, confirm appropriate placement by brief observation of bright red pulsatile blood emitting from the catheter hub, and cap the catheter.

5. If blood does not immediately flow into the needle

a. Pull out, reconfirm the landmarks, reposition, and try again.

b. Occasionally, the needle needs to be flushed of clogging tissue before reinsertion. Use a syringe of heparinized saline.

c. If the catheter cannot be placed in three attempts, try another site.

6. **When the catheter is successfully placed**
   a. Secure the catheter to the skin with suture.
   b. Obtain arterial blood samples as needed.
   c. Attach to manometer for continuous monitoring.
   d. Apply a sterile dressing.
7. **Document the procedure.**
8. **General considerations**
   a. Reassess daily the need for the arterial line.
   b. Confirm daily adequate blood flow to the lower extremity.
   c. If fever occurs, remember to draw blood for cultures from this site as well as from other indwelling sites.
   d. If the site remains clean, the catheter should be changed over a wire as needed.

■ COMPLICATIONS/PROBLEMS

1. Nonplacement of the line
2. Entry site infection
   The line must be removed and a new site used, if necessary.
3. Vessel thrombosis
   Transient occlusion is common, occurring in about 10% of placements. It is treated with removal of the line.
4. Suppurative thrombophlebitis
   This may require surgical drainage and IV antibiotics.
5. Distal ischemia
   Remove the line. Confirm distal pulses.
6. Bleeding from the placement site
   Be sure to check the connections. Under arterial pressures, a poor coupling of lines can result in rapid exsanguination. Occasionally, a stitch at the entry site will suffice.
7. Nonfunction

■ REMOVAL OF ARTERIAL LINES

1. Have a scissors or blade, gauze, and tape ready.
2. Always wear gloves when there is a potential for exposure to blood or other body fluids.
3. Remove sutures.
4. Remove the catheter.
5. Apply firm pressure at the entry site for 10 minutes (by the clock) and longer if the lumen was large or if the patient was anticoagulated.
6. After 10 minutes, confirm that bleeding has stopped.
7. Place a pressure dressing.
8. Check the site and confirm adequate blood flow to the extremity the next day.

15

INTRA-AORTIC BALLOON PUMP

The intra-aortic balloon pump (IABP) is used in settings of acute left ventricular failure. It may be used transiently after cardiac surgery or as a bridge to a definitive procedure such as transplantation.

■ INDICATIONS

1. Left ventricular failure
2. Inadequate perfusion (cardiogenic shock, myocardial infarction [MI], valvular disruption, weaning off cardiopulmonary bypass [CPB]).

■ CONTRAINDICATIONS

1. Any percutaneous approach to intravascular access is contraindicated in settings of skin lesions or infection overlying the site of insertion.
2. Aortic valve insufficiency
3. Aortic aneurysm

■ PRECAUTIONS

1. Coagulopathy
   Abnormalities in platelet count or function or in clotting factor concentrations should be corrected before insertion of the line.
2. Ongoing systemic infection
3. Dislodgment of these lines can result in rapid exsanguination.

■ EQUIPMENT NEEDED

1. Skin preparation supplies (iodine, chlorhexidine, or alcohol)
2. Local anesthetic (1% or 2% lidocaine, 25-gauge needle, 3-ml syringe)
3. Sterile gloves
4. Sterile towels or drapes
5. Supplies for Seldinger technique (or specific arterial line kit)

a. Needle (16 to 18 gauge)
b. 10-ml syringe
c. Guide wire
d. Scalpel
e. Dilator
f. Catheter
6. Supplies for IABP use
a. IABP
b. Balloon
c. Saline for lubricating the balloon
7. Heparinized saline in a pressurized delivery system
8. Blood gas syringe if needed for arterial blood sampling
9. Additional 5-ml syringe with heparinized saline
10. Suture for securing the catheter
11. Equipment for continuous monitoring of arterial pressure
12. Sterile dressing supplies

■ ANATOMY/APPROACH

Select the site.

1. Recall the orientation of the vessels in the groin.
   The artery is found halfway between the anterior iliac spine and the symphysis pubis (Fig. 15–1).
2. Palpate the groin to assess for adequate pulse.
3. Document the presence of distal pulses in the desired extremity.

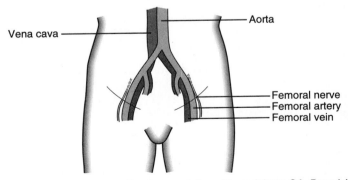

Figure 15–1 □ Anatomy of groin vasculature. (From Adams GA, Bresnick SD: On Call Surgery. Philadelphia, WB Saunders Co, 1997, p 239.)

■ ANESTHESIA

Local

■ TECHNIQUE (STERILE SELDINGER)

Most IABPs are available as part of established kits. Whenever possible, follow the instructions available with the specific kit. Also see Chapter 14.

1. **Prepare the patient.**
   a. Explain the procedure.
   b. Explain the risks and alternatives. Obtain consent if necessary.
   c. Answer any questions.
2. **Position the patient.**
   a. The patient must be supine.
   b. Raise the bed to a comfortable height.
   c. Confirm that all the equipment is available.
3. **Prepare the skin.**
   a. Use sterile technique.
   b. Prepare and drape the skin.
   c. Infiltrate the entry site with 1% to 2% lidocaine. Also infiltrate at the sites of anchoring sutures.
   d. Confirm that adequate anesthesia has been achieved. Infiltrate the areas where the sutures are likely to be placed as well as where the catheter is inserted.
4. **Insert the guide wire.**
   a. After confirming that adequate anesthesia has been achieved, locate the pulse with the index finger of your nondominant hand.
   b. An optional step is to nick the skin over the entry site with a sterile scalpel in order not to damage the catheter as it enters the skin.
   c. Place the 10-ml syringe on the needle and locate the pulse with the index finger of your nondominant hand.
   d. Insert the needle at a 45° angle to the artery (about 3 to 4 cm). Aspirate during insertion **and** withdrawal because often the vessel is encountered on the way out.
   e. When bright red blood pumps freely into the syringe, remove the syringe and immediately place your finger over the hub of the needle.
   f. Place the guide wire through the needle.
      Make sure that the wire passes **without resistance.** Remove the needle over the wire. Be sure to control the wire.
   g. Nick the skin at the entry site with a scalpel.
   h. Place the dilator over the wire and then remove.
      Watch for increased bleeding at the skin site. This is easily

controlled with gentle pressure. It may be necessary to dilate the skin wound slightly with a clamp.

5. If blood does not immediately flow into the needle

a. Pull out, reconfirm the landmarks, reposition, and try again. You may reposition 1 cm more superior on the groin.

b. Occasionally, the needle needs to be flushed of clogging tissue before reinsertion. Use a syringe of heparinized saline.

c. If the wire cannot be placed in three attempts, try another site.

6. Insert the balloon introducer.

a. Measure the length of catheter to be inserted. Estimate the length needed by measuring the distance from the insertion site to the sternal notch.

b. Wet the balloon with heparinized saline.

c. Remove the stylet from the introducer.

d. Place the balloon introducer over the wire into the wound.

e. Remove the wire.

f. Confirm the placement by aspiration.
   Flush with heparinized saline. Take care when flushing these lines to avoid air embolism.

g. Attach the lumens to the IABP and to the pressure monitoring system.

h. Secure the catheter in place by sutures.

i. Cover the entry site with a sterile dressing.

j. Confirm position by x-ray.
   The most proximal balloon tip should be 2 to 3 cm below the level of the left subclavian artery (Fig. 15–2).

7. Document the procedure.

8. General considerations

a. Reassess frequently the need for the IABP line.

b. Confirm daily adequate blood flow to the lower extremity.

■ **COMPLICATIONS/PROBLEMS**

1. Nonplacement of the line

2. Entry site infection
   The line must be removed and a new site used, if necessary.

3. Vessel thrombosis
   Transient occlusion is common, occurring in about 10% of placements. It is treated with removal of the line.

4. Suppurative thrombophlebitis
   This may require surgical drainage and IV antibiotics.

5. Distal ischemia due to occlusion or emboli
   Remove the line.

6. Bleeding from the placement site
   Be sure to check the connections. Under arterial pressures,

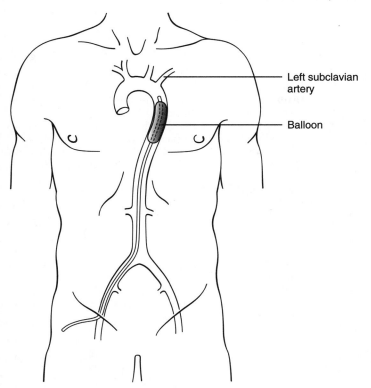

Left subclavian artery

Balloon

Figure 15–2 □ Appropriate positioning of IABP tip.

a poor coupling of lines can result in rapid exsanguination. Occasionally, a stitch at the entry site will suffice.

7. Nonfunction
8. Renal damage due to occlusion of renal arteries or hypotension

■ REMOVAL OF IABP

1. Confirm that IABP is no longer required.
2. Confirm that adequate IV and arterial access has been achieved if needed.
3. Have a scissors or blade, gauze, and tape ready.
4. Always wear gloves when there is a potential for exposure to blood or other body fluids.
5. Turn off the IABP.

6. Deflate the balloon by aspiration.
7. Remove sutures.
8. Pull the balloon out until it is just visible within the introducer.
9. Remove the balloon and introducer together with a firm continuous movement.
10. Apply firm pressure at the entry site.
    a. Hold above and below the catheter insertion site.
    b. Release pressure from the distal side first to allow some back bleeding to facilitate passage of distal blood clots.
    c. When no further clots pass, reapply pressure distally and release pressure form the proximal side to pass proximal clots.
    d. Reapply pressure over the puncture site for 30 minutes (by the clock).
11. After 30 minutes, place a pressure dressing or sandbag on the site.
12. The patient is to remain supine with leg extended for at least 6 hours.
13. Check the site and confirm adequate blood flow to the extremity at frequent intervals.
14. Evaluate the insertion site and distal perfusion in 24 hours.
15. If bleeding from the groin cannot be controlled with pressure, operative repair must be considered.

CENTRAL VENOUS LINES

□ □ □

These lines are use for hemodynamic lines (central venous pressure [CVP] or Swan-Ganz catheters), dialysis ports, and multiple lumen lines for prolonged medication or total parenteral nutrition (TPN) delivery. Venous blood sampling may also be possible through these sites.

□ **16** □

SUBCLAVIAN VEIN APPROACH

This is a common approach to central venous access. It is the most comfortable site for a conscious patient, an easy and relatively safe placement technique, and a very easy site to keep clean and protected. There is a higher risk of pneumothorax during placement of this line than during internal jugular or femoral lines.

■ INDICATIONS
1. Delivery of high concentrations of nutrition or medication
2. Delivery of inotropic medications
3. Prolonged delivery of medication
4. Hemodialysis
5. Hemodynamic monitoring of CVP

■ CONTRAINDICATIONS
1. Infection or lesion at the proposed insertion site
2. Thrombosis of the desired vessel

■ PRECAUTIONS
1. Coagulopathy
   Abnormalities in platelet count or function or in clotting factor concentrations should be corrected before insertion of the line.

2. Ongoing systemic infection

A peripheral site may be advisable until the source of infection is identified and suitable treatment has been begun. This may not always be possible.

■ EQUIPMENT NEEDED

There are specific kits available for many approaches. Refer to the instructions supplied with these kits for complete information.

1. Skin preparation supplies (iodine, chlorhexidine, or alcohol)
2. Local anesthetic (1% or 2% lidocaine, 25-gauge needle, 3-ml syringe)
3. Sterile gloves
4. Sterile towels or drapes
5. Supplies for Seldinger technique (or specific intravascular access kit)
   a. Needle (16 to 18 gauge)
   b. 10-ml syringe
   c. Guide wire
   d. Scalpel
   e. Dilator
   f. Catheter
6. If the Seldinger technique is not used, a catheter-over-needle system may be used.
7. Heparinized saline for flushing the catheter
8. Suture for securing the catheter
9. Equipment for continuous monitoring of central venous pressure, if desired
10. Sterile dressing supplies

■ ANATOMY/APPROACH

1. The subclavian vein is found anterior to the first rib and the anterior scalene muscle (Fig. 16–1).
2. The vein lies posterior to the clavicle, crosses under it medially and superiorly at the distal third of the clavicle, and joins the internal jugular vein at the base of the neck.
3. If right heart cannulation is desired, the left subclavian vein is more desirable to use than the right subclavian vein because it allows a smoother arc of the catheter once in place.
4. The most common approach is from an infraclavicular site, although it is possible to approach from a supraclavicular site.
5. Insertion site is generally from a point 1 cm inferior to the distal third of the clavicle (Fig. 16–2).

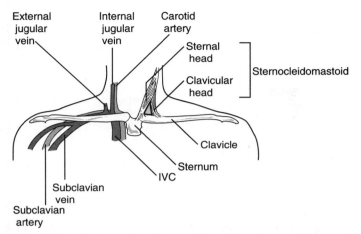

Figure 16–1 □ Anatomy of neck vasculature. (From Adams GA, Bresnick SD: On Call Surgery. Philadelphia, WB Saunders Co, 1997, p 242.)

■ ANESTHESIA

Local

■ TECHNIQUE (STERILE SELDINGER)

Kits have specific instructions.

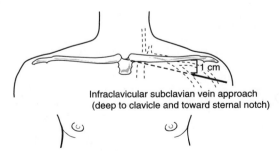

Figure 16–2 □ Needle entry site and directions for correct subclavian approach. (From Adams GA, Bresnick SD: On Call Surgery. Philadelphia, WB Saunders Co, 1997, p 242.)

1. **Prepare the patient.**
   a. Explain the procedure.
   b. Explain the risks and alternatives. Obtain consent if necessary.
   c. Answer any questions.
2. **Position the patient.**
   a. Supine and 15° Trendelenburg positioning will increase the venous filling of the subclavian vein.
   b. Elevate the bed to a comfortable height.
   c. Turn the patient's head away from the chosen site.
   d. Confirm that all the equipment is available.
   e. Place a roll under the spine between the shoulder blades (optional).
3. **Prepare the skin.**
   a. Use sterile technique.
   b. Prepare and drape the skin.
   c. Infiltrate the entry site with 1% to 2% lidocaine; then, infiltrate toward the clavicle. Once the clavicle is reached, march stepwise down the bone, infiltrating the periosteum.
   d. Estimate the length of catheter required to reach the superior vena cava (SVC) by placing the catheter on the sterile field and approximating its anatomic position after placement. It is often not necessary to insert the catheter to its hub.
4. **Insert the catheter.**
   a. Confirm that adequate anesthesia has been achieved.
   b. Place the 10-ml syringe on the needle.
   c. Insert the needle at a 20° to 30° angle to the skin. Direct the needle superiorly and medially toward the suprasternal notch (Fig. 16–3). Place a finger in the notch over the drapes to define this landmark (see Fig. 16–3A). Insert the needle just below the clavicle such that it is necessary to step down the bone to find the space beneath it. Advance along the dorsal surface of the bone and aspirate during insertion (about 5 cm).
   d. If the vessel is not encountered during insertion, slowly withdraw while aspirating because often the vessel is found on the way out.
   e. When dark venous blood flows freely into the syringe, remove the syringe from the needle. Immediately place your finger over the hub of the needle to avoid air embolus.
   f. Place the guide wire through the needle (see Fig. 16–3B). Ensure that the wire passes **without resistance.** Remove the needle over the wire. Be sure to control the wire.
   g. Nick the skin at the entry site with a scalpel (see Fig. 16–3C).
   h. Place the dilator over the wire and then remove. Watch for

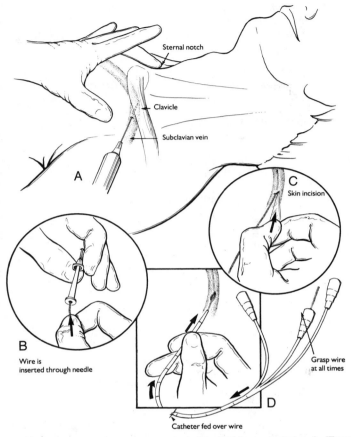

Figure 16–3 □ Subclavian vein cannulation (Seldinger technique). (From Dunmire SM, Paris PM: Atlas of Emergency Procedures. Philadelphia, WB Saunders Co, 1995, p 199.)

increased bleeding at the skin site. This is easily controlled with gentle pressure.

i. Place the catheter over the wire into the wound (see Fig. 16–3*D*).

j. Remove the wire, and confirm appropriate placement by aspiration of blood through each lumen, followed by flushing each lumen with heparinized saline, and cap the catheter.

5. **If blood does not immediately flow into the needle**
   a. Pull out, reconfirm landmarks, reposition, and try again.
   b. Occasionally, the needle needs to be flushed of clogging tissue before reinsertion. Use a syringe of heparinized saline.
   c. If the catheter cannot be placed in three attempts, try another site. It is wise to obtain an upright chest x-ray (CXR) before attempting to place the line on the opposite side. This evaluates for possible pneumothorax.
6. **If arterial blood is encountered**
   a. Remove the needle immediately. Discontinue the procedure.
   b. Obtain a stat upright CXR; repeat in 12 to 24 hours.
   c. Because of the anatomy of this site, pressure applied to the site may be inadequate to prevent bleeding (Fig. 16–4).
   d. Monitor the patient carefully for the next 24 hours for signs of respiratory distress or severe blood loss.
7. **If air is encountered**
   a. Remove the needle immediately. Discontinue the procedure.

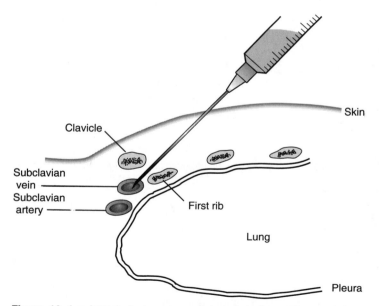

Figure 16–4 □ Intraclavicular approach to subclavian vein cannulation. (From Adams GA, Bresnick SD: On Call Surgery. Philadelphia, WB Saunders Co, 1997, p 244.)

  b. Obtain a stat upright CXR, PA and lateral. Repeat in 12 to 24 hours.
  c. Monitor the patient carefully for the next 24 hours for signs of pneumothorax.

8. When the catheter is successfully placed
  a. Secure the catheter to the skin with suture.
  b. Obtain blood samples as needed.
  c. Apply a sterile dressing.
  d. Obtain an upright CXR to confirm placement before infusion of fluids.
  e. Reposition as needed based on the CXR results.
  f. Attach to a manometer for continuous CVP monitoring, if desired.

9. Document the procedure.
10. General considerations
  a. Reassess daily the need for the central venous line.
  b. Check daily the site for infection.
  c. If fever occurs, remember to draw blood for cultures from this site as well as from other indwelling sites.
  d. If the site remains clean, the catheter should be changed over a wire every 3 to 7 days.

■ COMPLICATIONS/PROBLEMS

1. Venous air embolism
2. Pneumothorax
   a. Obtain a stat upright CXR to confirm the diagnosis.
   b. Place the patient on 100% O_2.
   c. If respiratory compromise is present, place a tube thoracostomy (see Chapter 29).
   d. This complication may occur up to 24 hours later.
3. Guide wire embolism
   Embolus must be removed by vascular surgery or interventional radiology personnel.
4. Arterial puncture
   Apply pressure at the puncture site. This site is difficult to compress.
5. Nonplacement of the line
   Obtain a CXR to rule out pneumothorax prior to considering attempting a line on the other side.
6. Misplacement of the line
7. Cardiac tamponade
   Remember Beck's triad: systemic hypotension, distended neck veins, muffled heart tones. This requires pericardiocentesis (see Chapter 31).

8. Entry site infection
    This requires removal of the line.
9. Vessel thrombosis
    This requires removal of the line.
10. Thrombophlebitis
11. Hemorrhage
    This may present as bleeding at the entry site, as an entry-site hematoma, or as bleeding into the mediastinum.
12. Nonfunction of the line

■ REMOVAL OF SUBCLAVIAN LINES

1. Ensure that the patient has no need for continued central venous access.
2. If a peripheral line is necessary, ensure that it is in place and patent.
3. Have a scissors or blade, gauze, and tape ready.
4. Always wear gloves when there is a potential for exposure to blood or other body fluids.
5. Place the patient in the supine position.
6. Clean around the catheter entry site with sterile soap if blood for culture is to be drawn.
7. Remove the sutures.
8. Remove the catheter.
    a. Remove all IV lines from the catheter.
    b. Clamp off or occlude all of the catheter ports.
    c. Have the patient hold his or her breath.
        This increases the intrathoracic pressure and decreases the risk of air embolism.
    d. Some long-term catheters have subcutaneous cuffs, which adhere to surrounding tissue (e.g., Hickman, Broviac).
        It will be necessary to break the adhesions between the subcutaneous tissues and the cuff. If the distance is short between the cuff and the skin insertion site, the adhesions may be broken using a hemostat inserted through the skin entry site. Be sure to use local anesthetic and clean the skin well. Occasionally a separate skin incision will be needed over the palpable portion of the cuff, and the adhesions should be broken through that incision. Occasionally the cuff will detach from the catheter with gentle pressure and may be safely left behind in the subcutaneous tissues.
    e. Remove the catheter with smooth, constant pressure.
    f. Confirm that the entire catheter has been removed.
        If a portion of the catheter breaks off during removal it may migrate to the heart and cause dysrhythmias or

respiratory difficulties. It must be removed by vascular surgery or interventional radiology personnel.

9. Apply firm pressure at the vein entry site for 10 minutes (by the clock) and longer if the lumen was large or the patient is anticoagulated.
10. Also apply light pressure to the skin entry site.
11. After 10 minutes, confirm that the bleeding has stopped.
12. Place an occlusive dressing for 24 to 48 hours.
13. Culture the catheter tip if clinically indicated.
14. Document the line removal.
15. Check the skin site the next day for evidence of infection or continued bleeding.

17

INTERNAL JUGULAR VEIN APPROACH

This is a common approach to central venous access. The line is not as comfortable as the subclavian line, but many operators believe that it is a simpler approach and that it may involve a lower incidence of pneumothorax during placement.

■ INDICATIONS

1. Delivery of high concentrations of nutrition or medication
2. Delivery of inotropic medications
3. Prolonged delivery of medication
4. Hemodialysis
5. Hemodynamic monitoring of CVP

■ CONTRAINDICATIONS

1. Infection or lesion at the proposed insertion site
2. Thrombosis of the desired vessel

■ PRECAUTIONS

1. Coagulopathy
   Abnormalities in platelet count or function or in clotting factor concentrations should be corrected before insertion of the line.
2. Ongoing systemic infection
   A peripheral site may be advisable until the source of infection is identified and suitable treatment has been begun. This may not always be possible.

■ EQUIPMENT NEEDED

There are specific kits available for many approaches. Refer to the instructions supplied with these kits for complete information.

1. Skin preparation supplies (iodine, chlorhexidine, or alcohol)
2. Local anesthetic (1% or 2% lidocaine, 25-gauge needle, 3-ml syringe)

3. Sterile gloves
4. Sterile drapes
5. Supplies for Seldinger technique (or specific intravascular access kit)
   a. Needle (16 to 18 gauge)
   b. Syringe (10 ml)
   c. Guide wire
   d. Scalpel
   e. Dilator
   f. Catheter
6. If the Seldinger technique is not used, a catheter-over-needle system may be used
7. Heparinized saline for flushing the catheter
8. Suture for securing the catheter
9. Equipment for continuous monitoring of central venous pressure, if desired

■ ANATOMY/APPROACH

1. The internal jugular vein exits the skull though the jugular foramen and runs posterior and lateral to the carotid artery. Both lie in the carotid sheath in the midcervical region (Fig. 17–1).
2. The vein runs medial to the sternocleidomastoid muscle at the

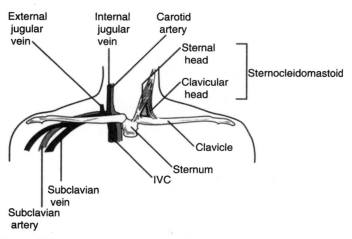

Figure 17–1 □ Anatomy of internal jugular vein. (From Adams GA, Bresnick SD: On Call Surgery. Philadelphia, WB Saunders Co, 1997, p 242.)

top of the neck and then passes under the muscle to join the subclavian vein behind the medial clavicle.

3. The path that defines the internal jugular vein may be traced between a point just anterior to the mastoid process and a point just lateral to the sternoclavicular joint.

4. At the base of the neck a triangle is defined by the two heads of the sternocleidomastoid muscle—medially by the sternal head and laterally by the clavicular head. The base of the triangle is defined by the medial clavicle. The internal jugular vein enters this triangle at the apex and runs lateral to the sternal head of the muscle.

5. The insertion site for the **middle or central approach** is at the apex of the triangle, aimed toward the ipsilateral nipple (Fig. 17–2).

6. The insertion site for the **posterior approach** is lateral to the sternocleidomastoid muscle starting 4 to 5 cm above the clavicle; the needle is inserted under the sternocleidomastoid muscle, aimed toward the suprasternal notch (see Fig. 17–2).

7. The approach from the right side has several advantages:

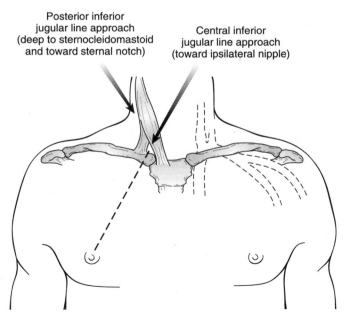

Posterior inferior
jugular line approach
(deep to sternocleidomastoid
and toward sternal notch)

Central inferior
jugular line approach
(toward ipsilateral nipple)

Figure 17–2 □ Insertion site for the middle or central approach is at the apex of the triangle, aiming toward the ipsilateral nipple. (Modified from Adams GA, Bresnick SD: On Call Surgery. Philadelphia, WB Saunders Co, 1997.)

a. It provides the straightest approach to the right atrium.
b. There is less of a chance of pneumothorax because the right pleural dome is somewhat lower than the left.
c. The right jugular vein is often larger than the left.
d. The position of the right jugular vein relative to the carotid artery is somewhat less variable than on the left.
e. There is no risk to the thoracic duct.

■ ANESTHESIA

Local

■ TECHNIQUE (STERILE SELDINGER)

The general steps are similar to the subclavian approach. Refer also to the placement of that line. Where steps differ, they are outlined here.

1. **Prepare the patient.**
   a. Explain the procedure.
   b. Explain the risks and alternatives. Obtain consent if necessary.
   c. Answer any questions.
2. **Position the patient.**
   a. The patient must be supine.
   b. Confirm that all the equipment is available.
   c. Pull the bed away from the wall. Ensure that it is at a comfortable height.
   d. Remove the patient's pillow.
   e. Remove the headboard of the bed if there is one.
   f. Turn the patient's head 30° away from the side of choice. Further rotation will defeat the purpose.
   g. From 10° to 15° of reverse Trendelenberg will facilitate engorgement of the veins.
3. **Prepare the skin.**
   a. Use sterile technique.
   b. Prepare and drape the skin. The drape may cover the face of the patient; ensure that the patient is comfortable and able to breathe.
   c. Infiltrate the entry site with 1% to 2% lidocaine. Also infiltrate over the sites of anchoring sutures.
   d. Confirm that adequate anesthesia has been achieved.
   e. Estimate the length of catheter required to reach the superior vena cava by placing the catheter on the sterile field and approximating its anatomic position after placement.
4. **Insert the catheter.**

a. Confirm that adequate anesthesia has been achieved.

b. Place the 10-ml syringe on the needle.

Often, a 22-gauge "finder" needle is used to sound for the jugular vein. The theory is that if the carotid artery is penetrated, the hole made is smaller than if a larger-gauge needle is used. The subsequent bleeding is less, and the risk of air embolism is less. Once the direction and depth of the jugular vein are determined, switch to the larger needle and proceed with the line placement.

c. With your nondominant hand, palpate the carotid pulse. You may feel comfortable putting gentle pressure medially on the carotid to retract it from the insertion site.

d. Insert the needle at a 20° to 30° angle to the skin.

   i. **Middle or central aproach** (thought to be the most reliable approach)

   Direct the needle inferiorly and laterally toward the nipple on the ipsilateral side (Fig. 17–3A). Aspirate during insertion (approximately 1 to 4 cm).

   ii. **Posterior approach**

   If the posterior approach is used, direct the needle inferiorly and anteriorly toward the suprasternal notch (approximately 5 cm) (Fig. 17–3B).

e. If the vessel is not encountered during insertion, slowly withdraw while aspirating because often the vessel is found on the way out.

f. When dark venous blood flows freely into the syringe, remove the syringe from the needle. Immediately place your finger over the hub of the needle to avoid air embolus.

g. Place the guide wire through the needle and complete the procedure according to the Seldinger technique (see Chapter 10).

5. **If blood does not immediately flow into the needle**

   a. Pull out, reconfirm landmarks, reposition, and try again.

   b. Occasionally, the needle needs to be flushed of clogging tissue before reinsertion. Use a syringe of sterile heparinized saline.

   c. If the catheter cannot be placed in three attempts, try the other side.

   d. Occasionally, when landmarks are not clear, a hand-held Doppler sonography may be used to locate the carotid artery and, thus, the jugular vein.

6. **If arterial blood is encountered**

   a. Remove the needle immediately. Discontinue the procedure.

   b. Hold pressure at the site for 10 minutes (by the clock).

   c. Obtain a stat upright chest x-ray (CXR) and repeat in 12 to 24 hours.

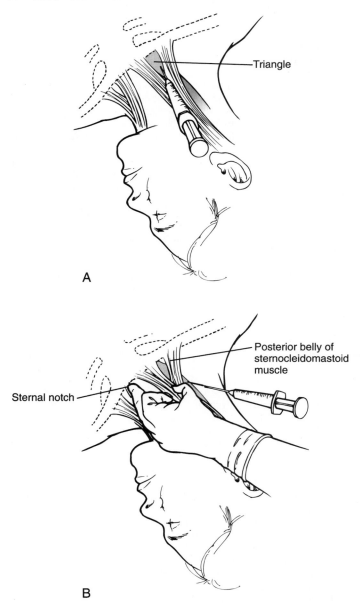

A

Triangle

Posterior belly of
sternocleidomastoid
muscle

Sternal notch

B

Figure 17–3 □ *See legend on opposite page*

    d. Once bleeding has been controlled locally, the procedure may be resumed.

    e. Monitor the patient carefully for the next 24 hours to watch for signs of respiratory distress or severe blood loss.

7. If air is encountered

    a. Remove the needle immediately. Discontinue the procedure.

    b. Obtain stat upright CXR, PA and lateral. Repeat in 12 to 24 hours.

    c. Monitor the patient carefully for the next 24 hours for signs of pneumothorax.

8. When the catheter is successfully placed

    a. Secure the catheter to the skin with suture.

    b. Obtain blood samples as needed.

    c. Apply a sterile dressing.

    d. Obtain an upright CXR to confirm placement before infusion of fluids.

    e. Reposition as needed based on the CXR results.

    f. Attach to a manometer for continuous central venous pressure monitoring, if desired.

9. Document the procedure.

10. General considerations

    a. Reassess daily the need for the central venous line.

    b. Check daily the site for infection.

    c. If fever occurs, remember to draw blood for cultures from this site as well as from other indwelling sites.

    d. If the site remains clean, the catheter should be changed over a wire every 3 to 7 days.

■ COMPLICATIONS/PROBLEMS

1. Venous air embolism
2. Pneumothorax

    a. Obtain a stat upright CXR to confirm the diagnosis.

    b. Place the patient on 100% O_2

    c. If respiratory compromise is present, place a tube thoracostomy (see Chapter 29).

    d. This complication may occur up to 24 hours later.

3. Guide wire embolism

Figure 17–3 □ Technique of internal jugular vein cannulation. Direct the needle inferiorly and laterally toward the nipple on the ipsilateral side. *A*, Middle approach; *B*, posterior approach. (Redrawn from Dunmire SM, Paris PM: Atlas of Emergency Procedures. Philadelphia, WB Saunders Co, 1995.)

Embolus must be removed by vascular surgery or interventional radiology personnel.

4. Carotid arterial puncture

   Apply pressure at the puncture site.

5. Nonplacement of the line

   Obtain a CXR to rule out pneumothorax prior to considering attempting a line on the other side.

6. Misplacement of the line

7. Cardiac tamponade

   Remember Beck's triad: systemic hypotension, distended neck veins, muffled heart tones. This requires pericardiocentesis (see Chapter 31).

8. Entry site infection

   This requires removal of the line.

9. Vessel thrombosis

   This requires removal of the line.

10. Thrombophlebitis

11. Hemorrhage

    This may present as bleeding at the entry site, as a neck hematoma, or as bleeding into the mediastinum.

12. Nonfunction of the line

■ REMOVAL OF INTERNAL JUGULAR LINES

1. Ensure that the patient has no need for continued central venous access.

2. If a peripheral line is necessary, ensure that it is in place and patent.

3. Have a scissors or blade, gauze, and tape ready.

4. Always wear gloves when there is a potential for exposure to blood or other body fluids.

5. Place the patient in the supine position.

6. Clean around the catheter entry site with sterile soap if blood for culture is to be drawn.

7. Remove the sutures.

8. Remove the catheter.

   a. Remove all IV lines from the catheter.

   b. Clamp off or occlude all of the catheter ports.

   c. Have the patient hold his or her breath.

      This increases the intrathoracic pressure and decreases the risk of air embolism.

   d. Some long-term catheters have subcutaneous cuffs, which adhere to surrounding tissue (e.g., Hickman, Broviac).

      It will be necessary to break the adhesions between the subcutaneous tissues and the cuff. If the distance is short between the cuff and the skin insertion site, the adhesions may be broken using a hemostat inserted through the skin entry site. Be sure to use local anesthetic and clean the skin well. Occasionally a separate skin incision will be needed over the palpable portion of the cuff, and the adhesions should be broken through that incision. Occasionally the cuff will detach from the catheter with gentle pressure and may be safely left behind in the subcutaneous tissues.

e. Remove the catheter with smooth, constant pressure.

f. Confirm that the entire catheter has been removed.

If a portion of the catheter breaks off during removal it may migrate to the heart and cause dysrhythmias or respiratory difficulties. It must be removed by vascular surgery or interventional radiology personnel.

9. Apply firm pressure at the vein entry site for 10 minutes (by the clock) and longer if the lumen was large or the patient is anticoagulated.

10. Also apply light pressure to the skin entry site.

11. After 10 minutes, confirm that the bleeding has stopped.

12. Place an occlusive dressing for 24 to 48 hours.

13. Culture the catheter tip if clinically indicated.

14. Document the line removal.

15. Check the skin site the next day for evidence of infection or continued bleeding.

18

FEMORAL VEIN APPROACH

This femoral vein approach is the easiest and safest line place-ment. The tip of the line will reside in the inferior vena cava (IVC); this is not a good placement for an ambulatory patient or one in whom pulmonary wedge pressures might need to be monitored. This line also has a higher site infection rate because of its placement in skin folds. Also, it is often hidden under bedding, and concerted effort is required to check the site for bleeding or infection.

■ INDICATIONS

1. Delivery of high concentrations of nutrition or medication
2. Delivery of inotropic medications
3. Prolonged delivery of medication
4. Hemodialysis
5. Hemodynamic monitoring of CVP

■ CONTRAINDICATIONS

1. Infection or lesion at the proposed insertion site
2. Thrombosis of the desired vessel

■ PRECAUTIONS

1. Coagulopathy
   Abnormalities in platelet count or function or in clotting factor concentrations should be corrected before insertion of the line.
2. Ongoing systemic infection
   A peripheral site may be advisable until the source of infec-tion is identified and suitable treatment has been begun. This may not always be possible.

■ EQUIPMENT NEEDED

There are specific kits available for many approaches. Refer to the instructions supplied with these kits for complete information.

1. Skin preparation supplies (iodine, chlorhexidine, or alcohol)
2. Local anesthetic (1% or 2% lidocaine, 25-gauge needle, 3-ml syringe)

3. Sterile gloves
4. Sterile towels or drapes
5. Supplies for Seldinger technique (or specific intravascular access kit)
   a. Needle (16 to 18 gauge)
   b. 10-ml syringe
   c. Guide wire
   d. Scalpel
   e. Dilator
   f. Catheter
6. If the Seldinger technique is not used, a catheter-over-needle system may be used.
7. Heparinized saline for flushing the catheter
8. Suture for securing the catheter
9. Equipment for continuous monitoring of central venous pressure, if desired
10. Sterile dressing supplies

■ ANATOMY/APPROACH

1. The vein is found halfway between the anterior iliac spine and the symphysis pubis.
2. Remember the orientation of the artery to the vein (NAVELS): nerve → artery → vein → empty space → lymphatics → symphysis pubis.
   (The vein resides between the pulse and the pubis; Fig. 18–1).

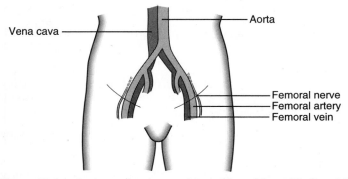

Vena cava

Aorta

Femoral nerve
Femoral artery
Femoral vein

Figure 18–1 □ Anatomy of groin vasculature. (From Adams GA, Bresnick SD: On Call Surgery. Philadelphia, WB Saunders Co, 1997, p 239.)

■ ANESTHESIA

Local

■ TECHNIQUE (STERILE SELDINGER)

The general steps are similar to the subclavian approach. Refer also to the placement of that line. Where steps differ, they are outlined here.

1. **Have all equipment ready.**
2. **Prepare the patient.**
3. **Select the site.**
4. **Position the patient.**
5. **Prepare the skin.**
   a. Use sterile technique.
   b. Prepare and drape the skin.
      Shaving may be necessary.
   c. Infiltrate the entry site with 1% to 2% lidocaine.
6. **Insert the catheter.**
   a. Confirm that adequate anesthesia has been achieved.
   b. Place the 10-ml syringe on the needle.
   c. With your nondominant hand, palpate the femoral pulse.
   d. Insert the needle at a 30° to 40° angle to the skin, medially to the pulse. Direct the needle superiorly. Aspirate during insertion (about 4 cm).
   e. If the vessel is not encountered during insertion, slowly withdraw while aspirating because often the vessel is found on the way out.
   f. When dark venous blood flows freely into the syringe, remove the syringe from the needle. Immediately place your finger over the hub of the needle to avoid air embolus.
   g. Place the guide wire through the needle and complete the procedure according to the Seldinger technique (see Chapter 10).
7. **If blood does not immediately flow into the needle**
   a. Pull out, reconfirm landmarks, reposition, and try again.
   b. Occasionally, the needle needs to be flushed of clogging tissue before reinsertion. Use a syringe of heparinized saline.
   c. If the catheter cannot be placed in three attempts, try the other side.
8. **If arterial blood is encountered**
   a. Remove the needle immediately. Discontinue the procedure.
   b. Hold pressure at the site for 10 minutes (by the clock).

  c. Once bleeding has been controlled locally, the procedure
     may be resumed.
 9. When the catheter is successfully placed
  a. Flush all lumens with heparinized saline.
  b. Secure the catheter to the skin with suture.
  c. Obtain blood samples as needed.
  d. Apply a sterile dressing.
  e. Chest x-ray (CXR) is not necessary before the use of this
     line.
10. Document the procedure.
11. General considerations
  a. Reassess daily the need for the central venous line.
  b. Check daily the site for infection.
  c. If fever occurs, remember to draw blood for cultures from
     this site as well as from other indwelling sites.
  d. If the site remains clean, the catheter should be changed
     over a wire every 3 to 7 days.

■ COMPLICATIONS/PROBLEMS

 1. Venous air embolism
 2. Guide wire embolism
    This must be removed by vascular surgery or interventional
    radiology personnel.
 3. Arterial puncture
    Apply pressure at the puncture site.
 4. Nonplacement of the line
 5. Misplacement of the line
 6. Entry site infection
    This requires removal of the line.
 7. Cardiac tamponade
    This may require pericardiocentesis (see Chapter 31).
 8. Entry site infection
    This requires removal of the line.
 9. Vessel thrombosis
    This requires removal of the line.
10. Thrombophlebitis
11. Hemorrhage
    This may present as bleeding at the entry site or internally,
    becoming a groin hematoma.
12. Nonfunction of the line

■ REMOVAL OF FEMORAL VENOUS LINES

 1. Ensure that the patient has no need for continued central
    venous access.

2. If a peripheral line is necessary, ensure that it is in place and patent.
3. Have a scissors or blade, gauze, and tape ready.
4. Always wear gloves when there is a potential for exposure to blood or other body fluids.
5. Place the patient in the supine position.
6. Clean around the catheter entry site with sterile soap if blood for culture is to be drawn.
7. Remove the sutures.
8. Remove the catheter.
   a. Remove all IV lines from the catheter.
   b. Clamp off or occlude all of the catheter ports.
   c. Remove the catheter with smooth, constant pressure.
   d. Confirm that the entire catheter has been removed.
      If a portion of the catheter breaks off during removal it may migrate to the heart and cause dysrhythmias or respiratory difficulties. It must be removed by vascular surgery or interventional radiology personnel.
9. Apply firm pressure at the vein entry site for 10 minutes (by the clock) and longer if the lumen was large or the patient is anticoagulated.
10. Also apply light pressure to the skin entry site.
11. After 10 minutes, confirm that the bleeding has stopped.
12. Place an occlusive dressing for 24 to 48 hours.
13. Culture the catheter tip if clinically indicated.
14. Document the line removal.
15. Check the skin site the next day for evidence of infection or continued bleeding.

19

PLACEMENT OF SWAN-GANZ CATHETERS

Swan-Ganz catheters are designed to provide simultaneous pressure readings from the pulmonary artery and the central venous system and to measure the pulmonary wedge pressure, which is an inference to the pressure of the left atrium. Cardiac output measurements may be made through thermodilution with these catheters.

■ INDICATIONS

1. Acute heart failure
2. Severe hypovolemia with requirement of rapid rehydration
3. Settings of extreme hemodynamic instability (sepsis, hemorrhage, pancreatitis, fluid shifts, cardiac disease)
4. Settings of extreme pulmonary disease such as adult respiratory distress syndrome
5. Blood sampling and cardiac output determinations

■ CONTRAINDICATIONS

1. Infection or lesion at the proposed insertion site
2. Thrombosis of the desired vessel

■ PRECAUTIONS

1. Coagulopathy
   Abnormalities in platelet count or function or in clotting factor concentrations should be corrected before insertion of the line.
2. Ongoing systemic infection

■ EQUIPMENT NEEDED

There are specific kits available for many approaches. Refer to the instructions supplied with these kits for complete information.

1. Skin preparation supplies (iodine, chlorhexidine, or alcohol)

2. Local anesthetic (1% or 2% lidocaine, 25-gauge needle, 3-ml syringe)
3. Sterile gloves
4. Sterile towels or drapes
5. Supplies for Seldinger technique (or specific intravascular access kit)
   a. Needle (16 to 18 gauge)
   b. Syringe (10 ml)
   c. Guide wire
   d. Scalpel
   e. Dilator
   f. Catheter
6. Supplies for placement of Swan-Ganz catheters
   a. Swan-Ganz catheter
   b. Appropriate monitor
   c. Protective sheath
   d. Syringe (3 ml)
7. Heparinized saline for flushing the catheter
8. Suture to secure the catheter
9. Sterile dressing supplies

■ ANATOMY/APPROACH

The catheter may be placed via any of the central venous approaches: subclavian vein, internal jugular vein, or femoral vein. The right internal jugular approach is the most direct route into the right atrium, although many operators prefer the left subclavian approach owing the more consistent gentle curve required to enter the pulmonary artery. The femoral approach is often difficult and may require fluoroscopic assistance. Please refer to the placements described for placement of the Swan-Ganz introducer.

■ ANESTHESIA

Local

■ TECHNIQUE (STERILE SELDINGER)

1. **Prepare the patient.**
   a. Explain the procedure.
   b. Explain the risks and alternatives. Obtain consent if necessary.
   c. Answer any questions.
2. **Position the patient.**

a. Supine and 15° Trendelenburg positioning will increase the venous filling of the subclavian or internal jugular veins. Supine and flat positioning is best if the femoral approach is used.
b. Elevate the bed to a comfortable height.
c. Turn the patient's head away from the chosen site (subclavian or internal jugular site).
d. Confirm that all the equipment is available.
e. Place a roll under the spine between the shoulder blades (subclavian site or internal jugular site).

3. Prepare the skin.
a. Use sterile technique.
b. Prepare and drape the skin.
c. Infiltrate the skin entry site.

4. Insert the introducer.
a. Confirm that adequate anesthesia has been achieved.
b. Place the 10-ml syringe on the needle.
c. Place the needle and guide wire according to the Seldinger technique. Ensure that the wire passes **without resistance.**
d. Nick the skin at the entry site with a scalpel.
e. Place the dilator over the wire, and then remove. Watch for increased bleeding at the skin site. This is easily controlled with gentle pressure.
f. Place the introducer over the wire into the wound.
g. Remove the wire, and confirm the appropriate placement by aspiration of blood, followed by flushing with normal saline or a heparin-containing solution.
h. Cap the introducer. **Confirm that the cap is well tightened,** because a large volume of blood may escape from the large lumen in a very short time.

5. When the introducer is successfully placed
a. Secure the catheter to the skin with one or more sutures.
b. Obtain blood samples as needed.
c. Prepare for placement of the Swan-Ganz catheter.

6. Prepare the catheter.
This procedure requires two individuals.
a. Flush each lumen with heparinized saline.
b. Check the integrity of the balloon by inflating with 1 to 1.5 ml of air.
c. Hook the pressure monitoring and infusion ports to the appropriate attachments.
   Note that many catheters must still be in the protective plastic container during the zeroing procedure; do not remove until the procedure is complete.
d. The sensitivity of the pressure monitoring may be tested by removing the catheter from the plastic container and moving the tip through space with a flick of your wrist.

An appropriate waveform should be visible on the monitor screen.

7. **Insert the catheter.**

This procedure requires two individuals.

a. When the catheter has been appropriately flushed and zeroed, it is safe to insert.

This is a two-person procedure; you will need a bedside caregiver who is experienced in the placement of these catheters. The caregiver will help by inflating and deflating the balloon for you during placement. Obtain additional experienced assistance if you are unfamiliar with the placement or use of a Swan-Ganz catheter.

b. Ensure that you have a large sterile work area on the bed on which the catheter may lie.

c. Ensure that the monitor is in clear view.

d. Place the catheter through the sheath protector. Move the protector to the very end of the catheter to keep it out of the way.

e. Under continuous monitoring, advance the catheter into the introducer into the superior vena cava (SVC) (internal jugular or subclavian approach).

f. When the tip of the catheter is clear of the introducer, inflate the balloon to 1 to 1.5 ml.

The balloon will allow the catheter to gently follow the flow of blood into the right atrium and through the heart.

g. Gently advance the catheter while watching the pressure monitor.

As the catheter tip passes from the SVC to the right atrium to the right ventricle to the pulmonary artery, you will notice the distinctive pressure readings (Fig. 19–1).

h. A wedged catheter will lose the pulsatile waveform and drop appreciably in pressure. When the catheter is wedged, deflate the balloon and confirm the return of pulsatile pulmonary artery pressures. Reinflate the balloon, and reconfirm the wedge position. If both of these criteria are met, the catheter is in a good position.

8. **If the catheter does not place easily**

a. Pull the catheter back and readvance.

Remember to deflate the balloon before pulling back on the catheter. It may take several attempts to adequately place the catheter.

b. The catheter may be stiffened as needed by flushing with 5 to 10 ml of cold saline.

c. The catheter may be slightly bent to facilitate an anatomic curve; take care not to kink or break any component of the catheter.

d. Occasionally, fluoroscopy is necessary for adequate placement.

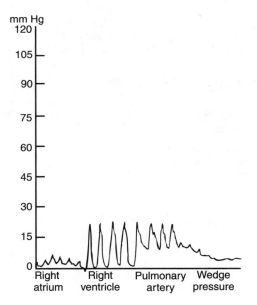

Figure 19–1 □ Pressure readings during advancement of the catheter. (Modified with permission from Shoemaker WC, Ayres S, Grenvik A, Holbrook PR, Thompson WL: Textbook of Critical Care, 2nd ed. Philadelphia, WB Saunders Co, 1989.)

9. **When the catheter is well placed**
   a. Make a recording of the appropriate pressures.
   b. Protect the external portion of the catheter by pulling the protective sheath over the catheter and attaching it to the introducer.
   c. Confirm that the introducer is well sutured and the caps are tight.
   d. Obtain a chest x-ray (CXR) to confirm placement.
10. **General considerations**
    a. Reassess daily the need for the Swan-Ganz catheter.
    b. Check daily the site for infection.
    c. If fever occurs, remember to draw blood for cultures from this site as well as from other indwelling sites.
    d. If the site remains clean, the catheter should be changed over a wire every 3 to 7 days.

■ COMPLICATIONS/PROBLEMS

The placement of a Swan-Ganz catheter may have the same complications or problems as other central venous lines, as well as the following:

1. Perforation of the pulmonary artery
2. Pulmonary infarction
3. Cardiac arrhythmias

■ REMOVAL OF SWAN-GANZ CATHETERS

1. Ensure that the patient has no need for continued pulmonary artery monitoring.
2. If a peripheral line is necessary, ensure that it is in place and patent.
3. Have a scissors or blade, gauze, and tape ready.
4. Always wear gloves when there is a potential for exposure to blood or other bodily fluids.
5. Place the patient in the supine position.
6. Remove the Swan-Ganz catheter.
   a. Ensure that the balloon is deflated.
   b. Remove the catheter a few centimeters at a time.
   c. Ensure that the catheter is intact on removal.
7. The introducer may be left in place as a source of venous access. If it is to be removed, remove it as you would any central venous catheter.
8. Clean around the catheter entry site with sterile soap if a culture sample is to be drawn.
9. Remove sutures.
10. Remove the introducer.
    a. Remove all IV lines from the introducer.

   b. Have the patient hold his or her breath. This increases the intrathoracic pressure and decreases the risk of air embolism.

   c. Confirm that the entire catheter has been removed.

11. Apply firm pressure at the vein entry site for 10 minutes (by the clock) and longer if the patient is anticoagulated. Also apply light pressure to the skin entry site.

12. After 10 minutes, confirm that bleeding has stopped. Place an occlusive dressing for 24 to 48 hours.

13. Culture the catheter tip if desired.

14. Document the removal.

15. Check the site the next day for evidence of infection or continued bleeding.

20

LONG ARM LINES

Alternatives to deep indwelling central lines are the percutaneous peripherally inserted central catheters (PICCs). The advantages to the use of these lines include ease of placement, decreased risk of pneumothorax with placement, and patient comfort.

■ INDICATIONS

Long-term venous access

■ CONTRAINDICATIONS

1. Infection or lesion at the proposed insertion site
2. Thrombosis of the desired vessel

■ PRECAUTIONS

1. Coagulopathy
   Abnormalities in platelet count or function or in clotting factor concentrations should be corrected before insertion of the line.
2. Ongoing systemic infection
   A peripheral site may be advisable until the source of infection is identified and suitable treatment has been begun. This may not always be possible.

■ EQUIPMENT NEEDED

Specific kits are available for placement of such lines. Follow the specific protocols associated with PICC lines. There usually are individuals who are specifically trained for the insertion, care, and removal of such lines.

■ ANATOMY/APPROACH

The basilic vein of the arm usually is used (Fig. 20–1), although the cephalic vein or the saphenous vein of the leg are possible options.

■ ANESTHESIA

Local

■ TECHNIQUE (STERILE)

1. **Prepare the patient.**
   a. Explain the procedure.
   b. Explain the risks and alternatives. Obtain consent if necessary.
   c. Answer any questions.
2. **Position the patient.**
   a. Place the patient supine.
   b. Elevate the bed to a comfortable height.
   c. Extend the arm laterally from the body.
   d. Confirm that all the equipment is available.
   e. Choose a vessel, usually the basilic vein (see Fig. 20–1).
3. **Estimate the length of the catheter.**
   a. Measure from the entry site of the catheter to the desired resting point of the tip. If the line is to be central, a resting point in the superior vena cava (SVC) above the level of the right atrium is appropriate.
   b. Some PICC line kits have a shielded region at the skin entry site for repositioning after placement. Before cutting the catheter, remember to leave about 8 cm of extra length to account for this.
   c. Always trim the catheter to result in a blunt end (straight across).
4. **Prepare the skin.**
   a. Use sterile technique.
   b. Prepare the skin.
   c. If the patient desires, consider infiltration of the entry site with 1% to 2% lidocaine.
5. **Apply the tourniquet.**
   a. Apply the tourniquet on the upper arm because this gives better dilation of the distal superficial venous system.
   b. Do not apply so tightly as to impair arterial flow into the extremity.

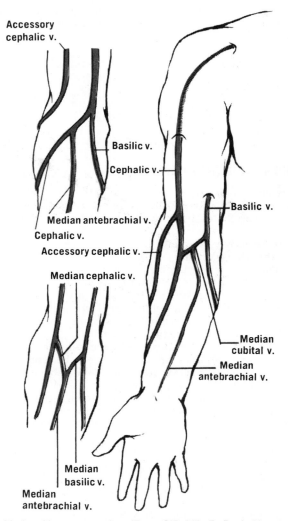

Figure 20–1 □ Upper arm veins. (From O'Rahilly R: Basic Human Anatomy: A Regional Study of Human Structure. Philadelphia, WB Saunders Co, 1983.)

6. **Insert the introducer.**
   a. Confirm that adequate anesthesia has been achieved (if used).
   b. Palpate the vein with the index finger of your nondominant hand. Apply gentle pressure to stretch the vein away from yourself.
   c. An optional step is to nick the skin over the entry site with a sterile scalpel in order not to damage the catheter as it enters the skin.
   d. Insert the needle and introducer at a 30° to 45° angle to the vein such that the tip of the catheter is more proximal to the heart than the hub.
   e. When dark venous blood pours freely into the catheter, hold the needle stationary.
   f. Remove the tourniquet.
   g. Remove the needle from the introducer.
7. **If blood does not immediately flow into the needle**
   a. Pull back but not completely out of the skin, reconfirm the landmarks, reposition, and try again.
   b. Occasionally, the needle needs to be flushed of clogging tissue before reinsertion. Use a syringe of heparinized saline.
   c. If the catheter cannot be placed in three attempts, try another site.
8. **Insert the catheter.**
   a. Insert the catheter through the introducer with smooth strokes.
   b. Position the protective shield so it covers the introducer.
   c. If the catheter kinks, a gentle pull-back and twist in the direction of the kink may help.
   d. To facilitate central placement, fully extend the arm to 90°, and rotate the patient's head to the side of insertion.
9. **When the catheter is successfully placed**
   a. Remove the protective shield.
   b. Retract and remove the introducer, taking care to maintain the catheter position.
   c. Remove guide wire, if used.
   d. Determine the patency of the catheter by aspirating for blood return.
   e. Flush the catheter with appropriate heparin solution.
   f. Secure the line to the skin with sutures. Place a sterile dressing.
   g. Confirm placement with x-ray.
   h. When placement is confirmed, attach tubing for delivery of appropriate IV fluid, if desired.
10. **Document the procedure.**
11. **General considerations**
   a. Reassess daily the need for the PICC line.

b. Check frequently the site for infection.
c. Patency of the line should be maintained by flushing with a solution of heparin (100 U/ml) every 12 hours. Use 1 ml per lumen.
d. Do not use syringes of less than 5 ml when flushing these catheters because they can generate sufficient pressure to rupture the PICC lumen.
e. If fever occurs, remember to draw blood for cultures from this site as well as from other indwelling sites.

■ COMPLICATIONS/PROBLEMS

1. Nonplacement of the line
2. Entry site infection
    This requires removal of the line.
3. Vessel thrombosis
    This requires removal of the line.
4. Suppurative thrombophlebitis
    This may require IV antibiotics and surgical drainage.
5. Catheter-related sepsis
6. Hemorrhage (usually minor)
7. Nonfunction

■ REMOVAL OF PICC LINES

1. Follow established institutional guidelines.
2. Make sure the patient no longer needs the PICC line.
3. Always wear gloves when there is a potential for exposure to blood or other body fluids.
4. Remove securing dressings.
5. Remove the catheter by grasping the catheter near the entry site and pulling 1 to 2 cm at a time. If resistance is met, apply a warm compress to the site and retry in 20 to 30 minutes. If resistance is still present, retape the line at its present site and retry in 12 to 24 hours.
6. When the catheter is completely removed, apply firm pressure at the entry site for 5 to 10 minutes and longer if the lumen was large or the patient is anticoagulated.
7. Confirm that bleeding has stopped.
8. Place a clean occlusive dressing for 24 to 48 hours.
9. Document the length of the removed segment.
10. Check the site the next day.

21

PERIPHERAL VENOUS LINES

The most common access is peripheral venous, and it is used for routine fluid replacement and medication delivery.

■ INDICATIONS

1. Requirement of IV fluid replacement for maintenance or rehydration purposes
2. Delivery of medication or nutrition

■ CONTRAINDICATIONS

1. Infection or lesion at the proposed insertion site
2. Thrombosis of the desired vessel

■ PRECAUTIONS

None

■ EQUIPMENT NEEDED

1. Skin preparation supplies (iodine, chlorhexidine, or alcohol)
2. Angiocatheter (18- to 22-gauge needles commonly used)
3. Heparinized saline for flushing the catheter
4. 10-ml syringe for flushing the catheter
5. Tape for securing the catheter
6. Local anesthetic (optional)
7. Nonsterile gloves
8. Sterile dressing supplies

■ ANATOMY/APPROACH

1. Most frequently, distal upper extremity sites are chosen.
   It is best to start more distally and then move proximally.
2. Palpable veins often are easier to cannulate than visible ones.
3. If no veins are apparent, try to warm the extremity, or place it in a dependent position to increase venous dilation.
4. In supine, nonambulatory patients, the lower extremity may be used.

5. Whenever possible, try to avoid sites that would be inconvenient to the patient.

These might include the dorsum of the patient's dominant hand, antecubital veins, or painful sites such as the volar surface of the forearm.

■ ANESTHESIA

None, or local may be used.

■ TECHNIQUE (CLEAN)

1. **Prepare the patient.**
   a. Explain the procedure.
      All needlesticks are painful.
   b. Explain the risks and alternatives.
   c. Answer any questions.
2. **Select the site.**
3. **Position the patient.**
   a. The patient should be comfortable, sitting or supine.
   b. Get a chair for yourself.
   c. Occasionally, armboards are required to immobilize sites such as the dorsum of the hand or the antecubital site.
   d. Confirm that all the equipment is available.
4. **Prepare the skin.**
   a. Use clean technique.
   b. Prepare the skin.
   c. If the patient desires, or if a large needle is to be used, consider infiltration of the entry site with 1% to 2% lidocaine.
5. **Apply the tourniquet.**
   a. Apply the tourniquet on the upper arm because this give better dilation of the distal superficial venous system.
   b. Do not apply so tightly as to impair arterial flow into the extremity.
6. **Insert the catheter.**
   a. Confirm that adequate anesthesia has been achieved (if used).
   b. Palpate the vein with the index finger of your nondominant hand. Apply gentle pressure to stretch the vein away from yourself.
   c. An optional step is to nick the skin over the entry site with a sterile scalpel in order not to damage the catheter as it enters the skin.
   d. Insert the angiocatheter at a 30° to 45° angle to the vein.

  e. When dark venous blood pours freely into the catheter, continue to advance the catheter slowly until the flow just stops.

  f. Back off slightly until the blood flows again, and advance the catheter over the needle into the vessel.

7. If blood does not immediately flow into the needle

  a. Pull back but not completely out of the skin, reconfirm the landmarks, reposition, and try again.

  b. Occasionally, the needle needs to be flushed of clogging tissue before reinsertion. Use a syringe of heparinized saline.

  c. If the catheter cannot be placed in three attempts, try another site. To avoid venous bleeding from the unsuccessful site, leave the catheter in the skin wound, and retry with a fresh angiocatheter. The unsuccessful angiocatheters may be removed later after the tourniquet is removed.

8. When the catheter is successfully placed

  a. Remember to remove the tourniquet.

  b. Secure the catheter to the skin with tape.

  c. Attach tubing for delivery of appropriate IV fluid.

9. Document the procedure.

■ COMPLICATIONS/PROBLEMS

1. Nonplacement of the line
2. Entry site infection
    This requires removal of the line.
3. Vessel thrombosis
    This requires removal of the line.
4. Suppurative thrombophlebitis
    This requires removal of the line.
5. Hemorrhage (usually minor)
6. Nonfunction

■ REMOVAL OF PERIPHERAL LINES

1. Make sure the patient no longer needs the IV site.
2. Always wear gloves when there is a potential for exposure to blood or other body fluids.
3. Remove securing tapes.
4. Remove the catheter.
5. Apply firm pressure at the entry site for 5 to 10 minutes and longer if the lumen was large or the patient is anticoagulated.
6. Confirm that bleeding has stopped.
7. Place a clean dressing.
8. Check the site the next day.

22

PERITONEAL TAP

The peritoneal tap is a very useful procedure for both diagnostic and therapeutic purposes. This procedure involves the placement of a sterile needle or catheter into the peritoneal cavity for the withdrawal of peritoneal fluid. The sampling of peritoneal fluid may be critical in determining a diagnosis for a patient with abdominal pathology. Furthermore, this procedure has several important therapeutic indications, especially in patients with respiratory compromise.

■ INDICATIONS

1. Various types of ascites
   a. Massive ascites
      Massive ascites increases intra-abdominal pressure and upward forces on the diaphragm. This may interfere with ventilation and is especially problematic for patients with concurrent pulmonary disease. These patients have little pulmonary reserve, and the increased intra-abdominal pressure may push them into respiratory arrest.
   b. Possible infected ascitic fluid
      Obtaining an abdominal fluid sample with sterile technique may help provide a diagnosis of peritonitis. Abdominal fluid may be evaluated with the use of Gram stains (for Gram-positive and Gram-negative bacteria), acid-fast stains (for mycobacteria), aerobic culture, and anaerobic culture.
   c. Possible malignant ascites
      Patients with known malignancy may develop new-onset ascites. This may represent liver failure, liver metastasis, or malignant ascites. Peritoneal tap may provide evidence of malignant cells. This finding greatly changes prognosis and treatment options for the affected patient.
   d. Chylous ascites
      This is a type of ascites in which free chyle (fatty fluid) collects in the abdominal cavity. This is an uncommon cause of ascites and is caused by either abdominal trauma or

lymphatic obstruction by tumor. Diagnosis and some relief of abdominal distention and pain may follow diagnostic or therapeutic peritoneal tap.

2. Blunt abdominal trauma

This is usually performed as a peritoneal lavage procedure.

3. Certain cases of acute abdomen when the decision concerning treatment is in doubt

An evaluation of peritoneal fluid may aid in diagnosis.

4. Acute pancreatitis in which serum amylase is not elevated

5. Primary peritonitis in infancy and childhood in which associated disease, such as cirrhosis or nephrosis, makes the risk of surgery prohibitive

■ CONTRAINDICATIONS

1. Coagulopathy

Patients with significant coagulopathies may not be good candidates for peritoneal tap. These patients may require fresh frozen plasma or platelets before any invasive procedures. Consult with your chief resident or attending physician in these cases.

2. Abdominal adhesions

The peritoneal tap procedure takes advantage of the fact that in the patient without intra-abdominal scar tissue, the abdominal viscera freely move in the abdominal cavity, bound only by their mesentaries. Thus, when a patient with significant ascites moves into the sitting position, leaning forward, the ascitic fluid collects in the anterior lower abdomen. It is generally safe to insert a needle into the anterior abdominal wall to retrieve fluid. However, in patients with previous abdominal surgery or infection, there may be scar adhesions. These adhesions may occur between the bowel and the anterior abdominal wall. The bowel is susceptible to injury if a peritoneal tap is performed on these patients.

3. Patient unable to hold still

For example, a patient with severe alcoholic intoxication is difficult to control, and iatrogenic injury to the bowel may occur if the patient moves suddenly during the procedure.

4. Patient with significantly distended bowel

If the bowel lumen is very distended, there is often high intraluminal pressure. A spinal needle that punctures distended bowel is more likely to cause luminal leakage.

■ PRECAUTIONS

1. Always use sterile technique. The introduction of bacterial infection into the peritoneal fluid of a patient may cause perito-

nitis and death. In addition, the contamination of a peritoneal fluid specimen may result in an incorrect diagnosis and unnecessary treatment.
2. In patients with previous abdominal surgery or infection, avoid inadvertent bowel perforation by performing peritoneal tap with the aid of ultrasound guidance.
3. Ensure that the bladder is decompressed before the abdominal tap. The patient should either void or be catheterized before the procedure.

■ EQUIPMENT NEEDED

There are specific kits available. Refer to the instructions supplied with these kits for complete information.

1. Local anesthetic (1% or 2% lidocaine, 25-gauge-needle [long] 3-ml syringe)
2. Spinal needle (20 gauge)
3. Syrine or vacuum bottle
4. Butterfly needle (at least 20 gauge with sterile tubing)
5. Povidone-iodine solution

■ ANATOMY/APPROACH

See the technique for each individual abdominal tap approach.

■ ANESTHESIA

Local

■ TECHNIQUE

There are two acceptable techniques for abdominal tap, which differ only in positioning of the patient.

Supine Position Abdominal Tap

1. Place the patient in the supine position.
2. Identify the flank region (Fig. 22–1).
    A flank tap is believed to increase the chances of a successful tap when small amounts of fluid are present. Other advantages of this site compared with low midline sites are the decreased chance for needling gas-filled loops of bowel and the decreased risk of needling the inferior epigastric vessels.
3. Avoid regions of previous surgical incisions.

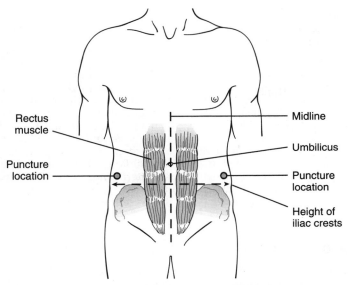

Figure 22–1 □ The flank region for peritoneal tap.

4. Prepare the skin with povidone-iodine solution and let the solution dry.
5. Put on sterile gloves. Using sterile technique and a 25-gauge needle, place a skin wheal of local anesthetic (preferably with epinephrine) over the site to be tapped. Advance the needle carefully and try to anesthetize the lower fascial levels and peritoneum.
6. Advance a 20-gauge spinal needle with the stylet attached until you feel the peritoneum "give." The stylet is removed, and a syringe of the desired volume is attached. If fluid is needed for diagnostic purposes only, a 10-ml syringe is adequate.
7. If fluid is to be drawn for therapeutic purposes, performing abdominal tap with the patient in the sitting position is easier.
8. When the tap procedure is completed, withdraw the needle, and place a sterile dry dressing over the site.

Sitting Position Abdominal Tap

For patients with significant ascites for which therapeutic tap is desired, it is often easier and more effective to have the patient sitting. The patient can lean forward and even support his or her upper body by placing the arms and elbows on a padded table. This leaning forward position allows the abdominal fluid to come inferiorly and anteriorly.

1. Perform steps 2 through 6 outlined above.

     For this technique, the flank is a good area to tap. Once peritoneal fluid is withdrawn with the syringe, a butterfly needle can be connected to the spinal needle. One side of a butterfly needle has clear plastic tubing that can connect to the spinal needle. The other end is the needle itself, and this can be used to puncture the seal on the vacuum bottle. The bottle will draw abdominal fluid out of the abdominal cavity and allow the removal of up to 1 liter of fluid per bottle. Additional bottles can be attached to the butterfly needle to allow the removal of additional abdominal fluid.

2. Place a sterile dressing when the procedure is completed.

■ COMPLICATIONS/PROBLEMS

1. Inability to withdraw fluid
   a. Little abdominal fluid is present
        If this is the case, try an abdominal tap with the patient sitting and leaning forward. This may be more effective than the supine position. Ultrasound is useful for localizing small fluid collections.
   b. Needle not passed into the abdominal cavity
        Be careful to slowly advance the needle so that you can feel the tissue layers as the needle is advanced. Once you feel a "pop" after passing through the muscle layers (in which there is more resistance), the needle tip should be in the abdominal cavity. If no fluid was encountered in your first pass, try again. If unsuccessful a second time, ask for help from a more experienced operator.
2. Puncture of the bowel
     It is quite safe to use a 20-gauge spinal needle, even if the bowel is inadvertently punctured. The hole will seal on its own. However, if ascitic fluid is inoculated with bacteria, the patient is at risk for bacterial peritonitis. Place the patient on appropriate antibiotic therapy if you have a high suspicion of bowel injury.
3. Stimulation of bleeding
     If you perform flank tap as described in this chapter, you minimize the risk of puncturing the inferior epigastric vessels. These vessels run from the groin region superiorly, to enter the rectus abdominis muscles laterally. These vessels then run under the rectus abdominis muscles toward the umbilicus. By

entering the abdominal cavity through a flank puncture, you are lateral to these vessels and other dominant vessels running in the abdominal wall.

If significant bleeding is encountered, pull out the abdominal tap needle and apply significant manual pressure on the abdominal wall for 10 minutes. Usually, bleeding stops without sequelae. In unusual cases, the patient will develop an abdominal wall hematoma.

23

PERITONEAL DIALYSIS ACCESS

Peritoneal dialysis access is an important technique used for patients with acute or chronic renal failure. The on-call physician is most likely to establish dialysis access for an acute indication. The technique is relatively simple and may be performed with local anesthesia. With the use of sterile technique, a peritoneal dialysis catheter is inserted into the peritoneal cavity and secured. Dialysis may be begun with low volumes shortly after the catheter is placed.

■ INDICATIONS

1. Acute renal failure
2. While a hemoaccess site is healing or maturing (e.g., arteriovenous fistula) or if hemodialysis is not tolerated
3. For intra-abdominal administration of chemotherapeutic agents (e.g., abdominal or hepatic malignancy)

■ CONTRAINDICATIONS

1. History of multiple previous abdominal operations
   This is a relative contraindication, superceded by the urgency of dialysis. Patients with an extensive history of prior surgery will likely have a great deal of scar tissue and adhesions, making it difficult to pass the peritoneal catheter into the pelvis.
2. Known abdominal adhesions or obliteration of abdominal space from infection
   With a previous abdominal infection, such as peritonitis, much of the potential space or abdominal dead space may be obliterated and scarred. This makes it difficult to pass the dialysis catheter safely.
3. Recent abdominal surgery
   Patients with recent abdominal surgery are susceptible to trauma from passage of the dialysis catheter. All patients with a bowel anastomosis or ligated structure are at risk for trauma.
4. Ileus
   Patients with an ileus will likely have dilated loops of small and large bowel. Any dilated structure, including the urinary bladder, is susceptible to iatrogenic injury. Unless the circumstances are dire, ensure that the abdominal ileus resolves and

that the urinary bladder is empty before beginning the dialysis catheter placement procedure.

5. Diaphragmatic tear

If there is a lack of integrity of the diaphragm, dialysate can move into the chest cavity and cause pulmonary or cardiac compromise.

6. Severe respiratory insufficiency

In these cases, the fluid dialysate creates increased intra-abdominal pressure, making ventilation more difficult.

7. Peritoneal malignancy

8. Large abdominal hernia

A lack of integrity of the abdominal wall makes it more likely that the dialysis catheter will not easily pass into the appropriate location in the pelvis. The catheter could end up in the hernia sac and cause soft tissue injury.

■ PRECAUTIONS

1. Use absolute sterile technique for all parts of the procedure.

The most common complication after catheter placement is infection.

2. Do not pass the dialysis catheter against resistance.

Patients who have had previous abdominal surgery will likely have adhesions and scar tissue between loops of bowel, omentum, peritoneum, and all other surfaces. Never force the catheter into the abdomen, because there is the possibility of perforating an abdominal or a pelvis viscus. If passage of the catheter meets resistance, redirect the catheter gently away from the resistance.

3. The urinary bladder should be empty before dialysis access is begun.

Have the patient completely void or place a Foley catheter before beginning the dialysis access procedure. It is not difficult to perforate the bladder if it is distended.

4. Exert extreme care if placing a dialysis catheter in a patient with dilated loops of bowel or a functional ileus.

Dilated viscera are more prone to injury during the passage of the dialysis catheter.

■ EQUIPMENT NEEDED

1. Skin preparation supplies, including sterile sponges and povidone-iodine solution
2. Sterile towels and drapes
3. Mask, sterile gown, and sterile gloves
4. Local anesthetic, preferably 1% lidocaine with 1:100,000 epi-

nephrine (be cautious in the use of epinephrine in patients with severe heart disease)
5. Syringe (5 or 10 ml)
6. Needles (21 gauge × 1½ inches and 25 gauge × ⅝ inch)
7. Sterile surgical instrument tray, including scalpels (No. 11 and No. 15), scissors, Kelly clamps, pickups, needle holders, sutures (2-0 silk, #1 and 4-0 Vicryl, and 4-0 nylon).
8. Peritoneal dialysis catheter with stylet
9. Dialysis tubing
10. Peritoneal dialysate
11. Dressing supplies, including sterile sponges, povidone-iodine ointment, and tape

■ ANATOMY/APPROACH

The basic structure of the anterior abdominal wall is important to understand. The paired rectus abdominis muscles lie on each side of the abdominal midline. Separating the two rectus muscles in the midline is a tendinous fascia known as the linea alba, is tough fibrous tissue and fascia. Lateral to the rectus muscles are the oblique muscles and fascia. This layer is thinner and easier to penetrate than the rectus muscles.

For the stylet technique described below, it is easiest to enter the abdominal cavity through the midline, piercing the linea alba (Fig. 23–1). For insertion of chronic dialysis catheters in which a muscle cuff is desired, an incision over a rectus abdominis muscle is preferable. For patients in whom acute peritoneal dialysis is desired and in whom midline scarring is present, an incision lateral to the rectus abdominis muscles is best.

■ ANESTHESIA

Performing this procedure with the patient under local anesthesia is preferable, because patient cooperation is helpful during

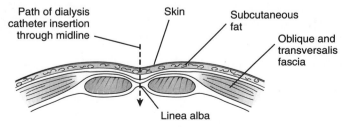

Figure 23–1 □ Cross-sectional anatomy for midline insertion of a dialysis catheter.

the procedure. For patients who are unable to tolerate local anesthesia, sedation, light general anesthesia, or both can be used.

■ TECHNIQUE

1. Shave, prepare, and drape the entire abdomen. The patient should be lying supine.
2. Administer the local anesthetic agent with a 25-gauge needle. Infiltrate the local anesthetic agent approximately 2 inches below the umbilicus in the midline. Be generous and administer at least 5 to 10 ml. First, infiltrate the skin with a large wheal. Then, infiltrate the deep subcutaneous tissues down to the peritoneum. The use of a local anesthetic agent with epinephrine minimizes bleeding and provides a longer local anesthetic effect.
3. Make a 5-mm incision vertically with the No. 11 blade just through the skin (Fig. 23–2). There should be very little bleeding in this plane. If the patient is uncomfortable, place more local anesthetic agent in the base of your incision. Wait a few minutes for the agent to take effect. Using the No. 15 blade, incise the fat and the underlying linea alba fascia, but do not enter the abdominal cavity.

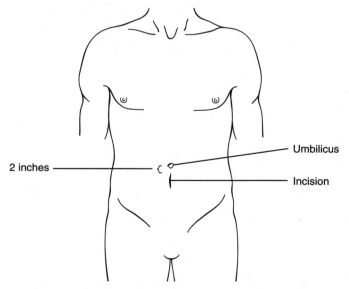

2 inches ──────────── Umbilicus

Incision

Figure 23–2 □ Incision made for midline insertion of a dialysis catheter.

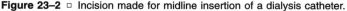

4. Place the peritoneal dialysis catheter with the attached stylet into the depth of the incision. Keep the catheter perpendicular to the abdominal wall at all times.

5. If the patient is awake, ask the patient to lift the head and tense the abdomen.

   This maneuver tightens the linea alba fascia, making it easier for the stylet to pass through if it was not cut earlier.

6. Insert the stylet and dialysis catheter into the abdomen. Always use two hands for this maneuver. One hand provides force, while the other hand holds the catheter to prevent excessive, sudden advancement of the catheter into the abdomen.

7. Once the peritoneal cavity is entered, direct the catheter toward the right or left iliac region.

   Advance the catheter without advancing the stylet; in other words, slide the catheter off the stylet. When the catheter has advanced and all catheter perforations are in the abdominal cavity, withdraw the stylet completely.

8. Use a syringe to gently aspirate the catheter.

   The return of peritoneal fluid confirms that the position is appropriate. In the absence of peritoneal fluid return, free irrigation of the catheter confirms the intraperitoneal position. A kidney, ureter, and bladder (KUB) x-ray is also helpful to document the position within the lower abdomen and pelvis.

9. Close the incision.

   If the deep fascia is visible and a defect is present, close the fascia with #1 Vicryl sutures. The skin can be closed with 4-0 Vicryl for a subcuticular dermal closure and with 4-0 nylon for skin closure.

10. Secure the catheter.

    Some catheters come with a fixation clamp, which clamps to the abdominal wall. We also recommend that the catheter be sutured to the skin with 2-0 silk sutures.

Special Circumstances

1. Long-term dialysis catheters such as Tenckhoff or Toronto Western catheters come with two cuffs (Fig. 23–3).

   These cuffs greatly decrease infection risk and provide longer life to dialysis catheters. These catheters are chosen when a patient is a candidate for long-term dialysis. For placement of these catheters, a paramedian incision is made so that one of the cuffs can be placed in the rectus abdominis muscle. A skin incision of 2 cm is made transversely, as shown in Figure 23–4. Direct vision of the dissection is critical. The rectus muscle is split, and the posterior rectus fascia and peritoneum are carefully penetrated. After the catheter is directed into the

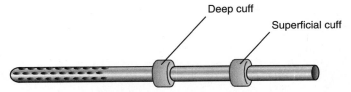

Figure 23–3 □ Straight double-cuff Tenckhoff catheter. The deep cuff lies in the rectus muscle, and the superficial cuff lies in the subcutaneous fat layer.

pelvis as described earlier, the deeper cuff of the catheter is placed in the plane of the rectus muscle. The second, or superficial, cuff is left in the subcutaneous tissue plane, and a tunnel is dissected above and lateral to the incision used for catheter placement (Fig. 23–5). The tunneling technique and the presence of two cuffs decrease infection risk because bacterial migration along the outside of the catheter is prevented.

2. If there is a midline scar and short-term dialysis is planned, make the incision lateral to the rectus muscles on either the right or the left side.

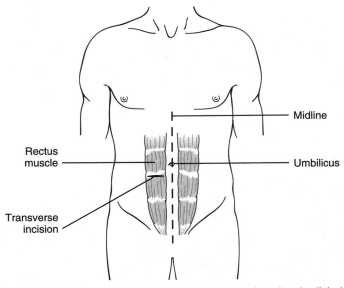

Figure 23–4 □ Transverse incision for placement of a chronic dialysis catheter.

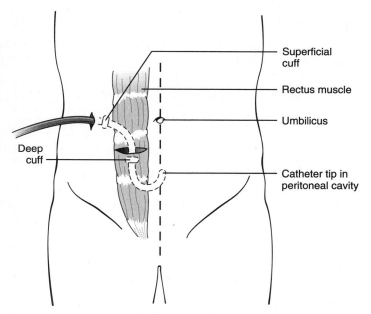

Figure 23–5 □ Double-cuff catheter placed through a transverse incision with the deep cuff in the rectus muscle. The superficial cuff is in the subcutaneous tunnel, and the catheter end is brought out of the lateral incision.

Avoidance of the midline is essential because these patients will likely have scar tissue and adhesions of viscera to the peritoneum. The use of an incision lateral to the rectus muscles is strategic because this minimizes the amount of tissue that the stylet must pass through when the catheter is placed.

■ COMPLICATIONS/PROBLEMS

Related to Surgical Placement of the Catheter

1. Intraperitoneal bleeding
   This complication is unusual but may represent a mesenteric or an omental vessel bleed. To minimize this risk, avoid advancing the stylet into the abdominal cavity.
2. Wound site bleeding
   This may be due to laceration of a branch of the superficial epigastric vessels. These bleeders usually stop on their own, but if they do not, suture ligation may be required.

3. Bladder perforation

   This complication is avoidable if the bladder is decompressed before beginning the procedure. A bladder laceration or perforation is best handled by a consulting urologist.

4. Bowel perforation

   This complication is avoidable if sites of surgical scars are avoided and the procedure is not performed in the presence of an ileus or a dilated bowel. Also, never advance the stylet into the abdominal cavity. The stylet is used to merely puncture the abdominal cavity. It is never pushed into the abdominal cavity after the puncture is made. Use care so that excessive force is not used when entering the abdominal cavity with the stylet. Inadvertent trauma can occur under these circumstances.

5. Leakage of dialysate

   If the entry made into the abdominal cavity is too large, leakage of dialysate fluid may occur with peritoneal dialysis. To avoid this problem, use care to minimize the size of the entry site through the peritoneum. If an open technique is used, such as with the placement of a long-term Tenckhoff catheter, ensure that the tissue layers are closed appropriately with sutures.

6. Hematoma formation and tunnel constriction

   If bleeding occurs with the placement of the catheter, a hematoma may form in the tunnel through which the soft catheter passes. This may constrict the catheter and prevent it from functioning.

7. Adynamic ileus

   An acute ileus almost always occurs after the placement of a dialysis catheter; it usually resolves in 24 to 48 hours.

Occurring After Placement

1. Peritoneal infection

   Peritoneal infection is the most common complication that occurs after the placement of a dialysis access catheter. Seventy-five percent of infections are due to Gram-positive bacteria, with the remainder of infections due to Gram-negative organisms. *Staphylococcus epidermidis* and *S. aureus* account for the majority of Gram-positive infections. The use of sterile technique at placement, frequent skin care and dressing changes, and aseptic handling of the catheter and tubing are required to lessen infection risk.

2. Catheter kinking

3. Catheter obstruction

   Omentum, loops of bowel, hematoma, and other physical obstructions can block flow in the catheter, requiring repositioning or replacement.

4. Dislodgement of the catheter

   Be sure to thoroughly secure the catheter to the skin to prevent dislodgement.
5. Hernia formation

   Although unusual, hernias can form at the site in which the deep fascia was transected and the abdominal wall weakened.

GASTROINTESTINAL TUBES

□ □ □

24

NASOGASTRIC TUBES

Adynamic ileus or intestinal obstruction can lead to the accumulation of gases and liquids in the gastrointestinal (GI) tract. Unless these are removed, a significant risk of aspiration is present. The placement of a nasogastric (NG) suction tube is used to decompress the proximal GI tract of gas and fluid.

■ INDICATIONS

1. Adynamic ileus
2. Small bowel or gastric outlet obstruction
3. Severe burns or polytrauma
4. After intestinal surgery with anastomosis
5. Gastric lavage for bleeding or poison ingestion

■ CONTRAINDICATIONS

Known or suspected facial fracture; the tube may be placed via the mouth

■ PRECAUTIONS

Known or suspected cervical spine injury

■ EQUIPMENT NEEDED

1. 16 to 18 Fr NG tube; these tubes may be sumped with a side arm port.
2. Lubricant jelly; K-Y jelly is sufficient, but lidocaine jelly may be used.
3. Topical nasal vasoconstrictors such as phenylephrine or cocaine (optional)
4. Topical anesthetic, such as Hurricaine spray (optional)
5. Emesis basin

6. Catheter tip syringe
7. Suction apparatus (i.e., wall suction or portable apparatus), tonsil tip suction tube
8. Gloves and eye protection
9. A small cup with water, with a straw for the patient to sip through
10. Benzoin and tape to secure the tube, once placed

■ ANATOMY/APPROACH

It is safer to place an NG tube in a conscious patient who can cooperate with the procedure. The risk of placement in an unconscious or a paralyzed patient is misplacement into the lungs.

■ ANESTHESIA

None, or topical lidocaine administered to the nares

■ TECHNIQUE (CLEAN)

1. **Prepare the patient.**
   a. Explain the procedure.
   b. Explain the risks and alternatives.
   c. Answer any questions.
2. **Position the patient.**
   Upright or decubitus, neck flexed
3. **Estimate the tube length.**
   Measure the distance from the patient's ear to the umbilicus; this is a good estimate of the needed length.
4. **Premedicate the patient.**
   a. Choose a nostril.
      Select the most patent one.
   b. Spray topical anesthetic to the back of the throat.
   c. Apply vasoconstrictor and topical anesthetic to the nasal mucosa.
   d. Apply lubricating jelly liberally to the tip of the tube and along the length of the tube as well.
5. **Have the suction apparatus turned on with the tonsil tip attached.**
6. **Insert the tube.**
   a. With the patient's neck flexed (confirm that there is no cervical spine injury), insert the tube into the nostril.
   b. Aim straight back toward the occiput.
   c. Apply firm, constant pressure to the tube.

   d. Have the patient hold the cup of water and take small sips and swallow as you apply pressure (Fig. 24–1).
   e. Continue to advance the tube to the desired length.
   A good guideline is to advance the tube until two black lines on the tube are visible out of the nares. The nose should be between the second and third black lines.
   f. Anticipate some gagging during placement.
   This may be decreased by spraying additional topical anesthetic to the back of the throat.
7. **If the tube does not pass easily**
   a. If the tube coils in the mouth or esophagus, chill the tube in some ice to stiffen it.
   b. If the tube does not pass at all, try the other nostril.
   c. If, during advancement, the patient begins to cough, withdraw immediately. This indicates misplacement into the lung.
8. **Once the tube is inserted**
   a. Hold it firmly in place close to the nostril; often, this requires steadying your hand against the patient's nose.

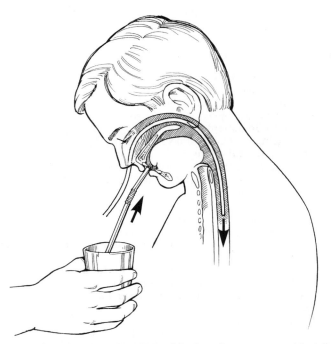

Figure 24–1 □ Position of patient while inserting a nasogastric tube. (From Rakel RE: Saunders Manual of Medical Practice. Philadelphia, WB Saunders Co, 1996, p 314.)

b. Attach the catheter tip syringe to the tube, and inject 30 to 60 ml of air into the tube. Listen over the epigastrium for the rumbling of the air into the stomach (Fig. 24–2).

c. Aspirate back on the syringe to confirm the efflux of gastric fluid. Normal stomach contents pH should be less than 5.

d. Secure the tube to the nose with benzoin and tape.

   Avoid taping the tube in such a way that pressure is applied to the nostril; this is a common cause of necrosis of the nares.

e. Be sure to tape the tube down to a second site, such as the patient's forehead or shoulder, so that inadvertent traction on the tube does not dislodge it.

f. Radiographic confirmation of the placement is not necessary if suction is to be applied.

   The tube may be used for decompression immediately. NG tubes have radio-opaque marker tape incorporated into their design so they are visible on routine abdominal x-ray.

g. You may want to place a mark on the tube near the nose, to mark proper placement.

9. Document the procedure.

10. Routine care

a. Record suction output volume and character.

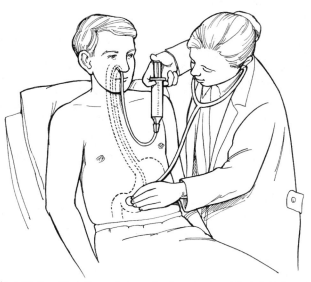

Figure 24–2 □ Technique for confirming nasogastric tube placement. (From Rakel RE: Saunders Manual of Medical Practice. Philadelphia, WB Saunders Co, 1996, p 314.)

b. If the output is of a large volume, consider replacement of NG output: use 0.5 to 1 ml lactated Ringer's or normal saline (NS) + 30 mEq KCl/L per ml of output; replace intravenously each shift.

c. If the tube becomes blocked, attempt to irrigate it with 30 to 40 ml of NS.

   If the block does not resolve, reposition the tube. Check with the nursing staff to see whether there are protocols regarding routine irrigation of NG tubes. If not, have the tube routinely irrigated at least every shift and PRN with 30 to 40 ml of NS.

d. If routine x-rays are taken for other reasons, examine them for appropriate placement of the NG tube.

e. An indwelling NG tube often is very uncomfortable.

   Make sure the patient has some throat lozenges at the bedside for PRN use.

■ COMPLICATIONS/PROBLEMS

1. Aspiration pneumonia
2. Trauma to nasal mucosa or nares skin
3. Trauma to lung or esophagus
4. Sinusitis

   Indwelling catheters can cause trauma and swelling around sinus orifices, leading to acute sinusitis. Think of this as a possible cause of fever in a patient with an NG tube.

5. Nonfunctional or blocked tube

   Various techniques are useful to unclog NG tubes.

   a. Often, simply disconnecting the tube from the suction and reattaching it are sufficient to encourage function.

   b. If the tube has a vent port (Salem sump or Anderson tube), inject a small amount of air into this port.

      When functioning normally, the port will make a hissing sound.

   c. Flush the tube with a small volume of NS. Use a catheter tip syringe.

   d. Reposition the tube if it is too far in or too far out.

6. Dislodged tube

   a. A tube that is placed too low (i.e., past the pylorus) will drain large volumes of bile.

      This may be confirmed by an abdominal x-ray. If the tube is too low, reposition the tube back into the stomach.

   b. A tube that is placed too high (i.e., in the esophagus) will not adequately drain the stomach and increases the risk of aspiration.

Reposition the tube and confirm its placement with an injection of air.

7. Trauma to the gastric mucosa

■ REMOVAL

1. Confirm that the tube is no longer necessary.
2. Wear gloves and eyewear to protect yourself from exposure to secretions.
3. Remove the tube from suction.
4. Remove the securing tape from the patient.
5. Hand the patient a tissue because he or she will want to blow the nose.
6. Remove the tube with a steady pressure.
7. Discard in appropriate receptacle.

25

FEEDING TUBES

Enteral feeding is preferable to parenteral nutrition. The use of the gut is physiological and decreases the risk of translocation of intraluminal bacteria, which may be a septic source. In addition, there are none of the complications of IV lines.

The tubes used for feeding are smaller and more flexible than the tubes used for nasogastric (NG) drainage. Their placement is identical to that of NG tubes except that the ultimate placement may be in the duodenum or jejunum and often a guide wire is used for placement. These tubes are too soft to be used for NG suction.

■ INDICATIONS

Enteral feeding and delivery of medication

■ CONTRAINDICATIONS

1. Known or suspected facial fracture
2. Adynamic ileus
3. Malabsorptive syndromes
4. Intestinal obstruction

■ PRECAUTIONS

1. Known or suspected cervical spine injury
2. Gastroenteritis

■ EQUIPMENT NEEDED

1. Feeding tube
2. Lubricant jelly; K-Y jelly is sufficient, but lidocaine jelly may be used
3. Topical nasal vasoconstrictors, such as phenylephrine or cocaine (optional)
4. Topical anesthetic, such as Hurricaine spray (optional)
5. Emesis basin
6. Catheter tip syringe

7. Suction apparatus (i.e., wall suction or portable apparatus), tonsil tip suction tube
8. Gloves and eye protection
9. A small cup with water, with a straw for the patient to sip through
10. Benzoin and tape to secure the tube, once placed

■ ANATOMY/APPROACH

The placement of feeding tubes is very similar to that of NG tubes, but because they are thinner and more flexible, these tubes often are more difficult to place. It is not uncommon to require pharmacological or fluoroscopic assistance in their positioning. In addition, it is advisable to confirm the placement of these tubes by x-ray before use.

■ ANESTHESIA

None, or topical lidocaine administered to the nares

■ TECHNIQUE

1. **Follow the procedure for placement of an NG tube in Chapter 24.**
   If the tube has a guide wire, leave this in place until the confirmatory x-ray is taken.
2. **If duodenal or jejunal placement is desired**
   a. Consider the use of a weighted tube.
   b. Insert to an additional 20 to 40 cm of length.
   c. Place the patient onto the right side for 8 to 12 hours.
   d. When appropriately placed, fluid aspirates should have a pH of more than 7.
   e. Confirm placement by abdominal x-ray (kidney, ureter, bladder [KUB]).
3. **The following substances can be used to increase stomach motility to encourage passage**
   a. Metoclopramide
   b. Cisapride
   c. Erythromycin
4. **If the above steps fail to pass the tube from the stomach to the duodenum, use fluoroscopy to place the tube under direct vision.**
5. **Confirm placement with an abdominal x-ray.**
   Only then is it safe to feed.
6. **Document the procedure.**

■ COMPLICATIONS/PROBLEMS OF FEEDING TUBES

1. Aspiration pneumonia

   This may be due to tube misplacement or reflux. Direct delivery of formula to the lungs can cause a profound chemical pneumonitis.
2. Trauma to nasal mucosa or nares skin
3. Trauma to lung or esophagus
4. Sinusitis

   Indwelling catheters can cause trauma and swelling around sinus orifices, leading to acute sinusitis. Think of this as a possible cause of fever in a patient with a feeding tube.
5. Blocked tube

   Often, the formula that is used in tube feedings will clog the tube. Various techniques are useful to unclog feeding tubes.
   a. Flush the tube with a small volume of saline.

      Use a small syringe because this can generate a greater pressure.
   b. If saline is ineffective, hot water or carbonated soda may be used.
   c. A slurry of pancreatic enzymes and bicarbonate also may be used.
6. Dislodged tube

   Misplacement of a feeding tube may be identified by radiography, or it may become evident by feeding intolerance. Reposition based on the x-ray.
7. Perforation of intestines.

■ REMOVAL OF FEEDING TUBES

1. Confirm that the tube is no longer necessary.
2. Wear gloves and eyewear to protect yourself from exposure to secretions.
3. Remove the tube from the infusion pump.
4. Remove the securing tape from the patient.
5. Hand the patient a tissue because he or she will want to blow the nose.
6. Remove the tube with a steady pressure.

26

REPLACEMENT OF GASTROSTOMY TUBES

Feeding gastrostomy tubes can be placed endoscopically or by an open surgical approach. These tubes enter through a stoma in the anterior abdominal wall and through a hole in the stomach. They may be held in place by an internal balloon or flange, or they may be sutured at the skin level. On occasion, these may become dislodged and require replacement.

■ INDICATIONS

Continued need for enteral feeding through a gastrostomy tube

■ PRECAUTIONS

1. A tube placed within the past 6 weeks will have an immature tract, and replacement can disrupt the junction between the stomach and the anterior abdominal wall. This results in placement of the tube into the peritoneum and not into the stomach, leading to peritonitis on resumption of feeding.
2. Active infection around the gastrostomy site may make the replacement difficult or uncomfortable.
3. A tube that has been dislodged for more than 24 hours may be impossible to pass.

■ EQUIPMENT NEEDED

1. An appropriate-sized tube or Foley catheter; have available a tube the size of the one that came out and one that is one size smaller
2. Water-soluble lubricant

■ ANESTHESIA

None required

■ TECHNIQUE (CLEAN)

1. **Lubricate the tip of the tube with water-soluble lubricant (K-Y jelly).**

2. **Insert the tube into the stoma with gentle consistent pressure. DO NOT FORCE.**
3. **If the tube passes easily, inflate the balloon with normal saline (NS).**
4. **Confirm placement of the tube.**
   a. If the tract is less than 6 weeks old, inject a small amount of water-soluble contrast medium through the catheter, and obtain an abdominal x-ray to confirm the passage of dye into the stomach before use of the tube.
   b. If the tract is well established, aspiration of gastric contents and injection of a small amount of air into the tube while listening over the epigastrium should be sufficient.
5. **If the tube does not pass easily**
   a. Try a smaller tube.
   b. On occasion, interventional radiologists are able to pass a wire through a narrow tract and dilate the tract in a procedure similar to the Seldinger technique.
6. **Document the procedure.**

■ COMPLICATIONS/PROBLEMS

1. Misplacement of the tube
   Peritonitis may result if the tube is used.
2. Loss of the tract
   This is especially likely if the tube has been left out for longer than 24 hours.

■ REMOVAL OF GASTROSTOMY TUBES

1. Confirm that the gastrostomy tube is no longer needed.
2. Deflate the balloon, if present.
3. Remove the catheter with a slow, consistent pressure.
4. Place a simple gauze dressing on the site. Change the dressing daily until the gastrostomy closes. This should close within 24 to 72 hours. Occasionally, the tract stays patent and will require surgical closure.

27

SENGSTAKEN-BLAKEMORE TUBES

A Sengstaken-Blakemore tube may be used to tamponade active bleeding from documented esophageal or gastric varices. It may be placed after unsuccessful attempts at endoscopic injection or cautery, or it may be used while awaiting endoscopy or definitive surgical therapy.

■ INDICATIONS

Active massive bleeding from known esophageal or gastric varices unresponsive to vasopressin or endoscopic sclerosing therapy

■ PRECAUTIONS

1. Make sure that the patient has adequate IV access and is well resuscitated.
2. Placement of an esophageal/gastric tamponade tube is a high-risk procedure. Transfer the patient to the intensive care unit (ICU) and monitor appropriately.
3. Control of the airway with endotracheal intubation is strongly recommended.

■ EQUIPMENT NEEDED

1. Sengstaken-Blakemore tube (Fig. 27–1)
2. Suction apparatus
3. 60-ml syringe
4. Electrocardiogram (ECG) and SaO_2 monitoring
5. O_2, if required
6. Pressure manometer
7. Water-soluble lubrication or 2% lidocaine jelly
8. Nasogastric (NG) tube
9. Gloves and eye protection
10. Hemostat clamps (2)
11. Scissors or scalpel at the bedside
12. Normal saline (NS) or water-soluble contrast material for filling the balloons.

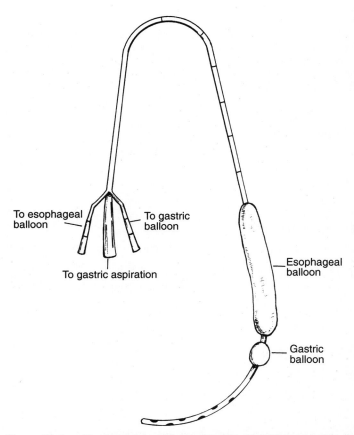

To esophageal balloon

To gastric balloon

To gastric aspiration

Esophageal balloon

Gastric balloon

Figure 27–1 □ The Sengstaken-Blakemore tube. The Minnesota tube is similar; it has an additional port for esophageal aspiration. (From Marshall SA, Ruedy J: On Call Principles and Protocols, 2nd ed. Philadelphia, WB Saunders Co, 1993, p 102.)

■ ANATOMY/APPROACH

Position the patient in left lateral decubitus or supine position.

■ ANESTHESIA

None, or topical lidocaine administered to the nares

■ TECHNIQUE

1. **Prepare the patient.**
   a. Explain the procedure.
   b. Explain the risks and alternatives. Obtain consent if necessary.
   c. Answer any questions.
2. **Position of the patient**
   Left lateral decubitus or supine, neck flexed
3. **Empty the stomach.**
   This may be done with the existing NG tube, if placed.
4. **Premedicate the patient (optional).**
   a. Choose a nostril; select the most patent one.
   b. Spray topical anesthetic to the back of the throat.
   c. Apply vasoconstrictor and topical anesthetic to the nasal mucosa.
   d. Apply lubricating jelly liberally to the tip of the tube and along the length of the tube.
5. **Have the suction apparatus turned on with the tonsil tip attached.**
6. **Test the balloons on the tube.**
7. **Insert the tube.**
   a. With the patient's neck flexed, insert the tube into the nostril.
   b. Aim straight back toward the occiput.
   c. Have the patient swallow, if possible.
   d. Continue to advance the tube to 45 to 50 cm.
8. **If the tube does not pass easily**
   a. If the tube coils in the mouth or esophagus, chill the tube in some ice to stiffen it.
   b. If the tube does not pass at all, try the other nostril.
   c. If, during advancement, the patient begins to cough, withdraw immediately. This indicates misplacement into the trachea.
9. **Inflate the gastric balloon.**
   a. This may take 100 to 250 ml of NS, or a dilute solution of contrast material may be used.

Stop inflating the tube immediately if the patient complains of pain or fullness in the esophagus during inflation.

b. Attach the catheter-tip syringe to the tube and inject 30 to 60 ml of air into the tube. Listen over the epigastrium for the rumbling of the air into the stomach.

c. Aspirate back on the syringe to confirm the efflux of blood or gastric fluid. pH should be less than 5.

d. Clamp the tube.

10. **Apply gentle traction on the tube.**
    This pulls the gastric balloon up to the gastroesophageal junction.

11. **Secure the tube to the face or to a helmet with a face mask.**
    If the tube is attached directly to the patient's face, pad it well.

12. **Pass a regular NG tube through the other nostril.**
    This is placed to remove oral secretions that are swallowed. This tube is placed to low continuous suction.

13. **Irrigate through the tubes.**
    a. Irrigate through both the esophageal NG tube and the distal port of the Sengstaken-Blakemore tube.
    b. If the bleeding has stopped, it may not be necessary to inflate the esophageal balloon. Reconfirm this on several occasions during the first few hours of therapy.
    c. If continued bleeding is noted:

14. **Inflate the esophageal balloon to 35 to 40 mm Hg.**

15. **Confirm placement with a chest x-ray.**
    The final position is diagrammed in Figure 27–2.

16. **Document the procedure.**

17. **Provide routine care.**
    a. Maintain continuous suction on the esophageal NG tube.
    b. Maintain the tube in place for up to 24 hours if effective. Deflate the balloons every 4 to 6 hours to confirm the continued need of the tube and to avoid ischemia of the gastric or esophageal mucosa.

■ COMPLICATIONS/PROBLEMS

1. Continued hemorrhage
2. Esophageal or gastric rupture
3. Esophageal or gastric erosion
4. Aspiration of inadequately drained esophageal secretions
5. Airway obstruction

■ MANAGEMENT/FOLLOW-UP/REMOVAL

1. Confirm that the tube is no longer needed.
2. Deflate the esophageal balloon.

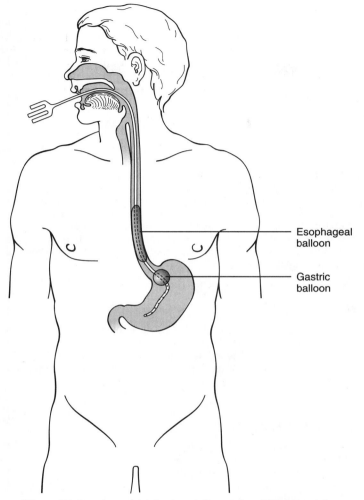

Figure 27–2 □ Appropriately placed Sengstaken-Blakemore tube.

3. One hour later, deflate the gastric balloon.
4. Leave the tube in place and irrigate the gastric tube every 30 minutes for 1 to 2 hours to confirm cessation of bleeding.
5. If bleeding has stopped, the tube may be removed.

NEUROLOGIC PROCEDURES

□ □ □

.⏐28⏐.

LUMBAR PUNCTURE

Lumbar puncture is an important technique that is commonly performed while on call. It is most frequently used as a diagnostic procedure to identify infectious processes of the central nervous system. Occasionally, the on-call physician will perform lumbar puncture to administer diagnostic or therapeutic agents. The procedure is relatively simple to perform and is used routinely in working up children with sepsis or adults with fever and mental status changes.

■ INDICATIONS

1. To obtain cerebrospinal fluid (CSF) for the diagnosis of infectious, inflammatory, or neoplastic disease
2. To administer diagnostic and therapeutic agents and drugs
3. To treat hydrocephalus for selective patients (performed by neurosurgeon)

■ CONTRAINDICATIONS

1. Increased intracranial pressure
2. Intracranial mass or mass effect
3. Anticoagulation or bleeding dysfunction
4. Soft tissue infection adjacent to planned puncture site or spinal osteomyelitis

■ PRECAUTIONS

1. Whenever possible, avoid spinal tap in patients on anticoagulants or who have bleeding tendencies.
   Patients with renal failure, von Willebrand's disease, thrombocytopenia, hemophilia, and liver disease carry a high risk of bleeding with spinal tap procedures. Bleeding into the CSF

space can cause an array of neurologic problems and complications.

2. Always rule out a mass lesion before performing a spinal tap whenever papilledema or other signs of increased intracranial pressure are present.

   A computed tomography scan is appropriate in these instances. If CSF is removed below a site of neural tissue edema, a downward pressure gradient may form, causing herniation and possibly death.

3. Be careful to always use aseptic technique and care when performing spinal tap.

   One can accidently introduce organisms into the subarachnoid space during the procedure, which can cause meningitis or an epidural or a subdural empyema.

4. In elderly patients, withdraw CSF slowly and withdraw only the amount of fluid that is needed.

   The removal of a large volume of CSF or rapid withdrawal can cause tearing of fragile perforating veins and a subdural hematoma.

5. If a dry tap occurs, the needle may be too lateral or too deep. Withdraw the needle, review the landmarks, and carefully repeat the tap.

■ EQUIPMENT NEEDED

Prepared kits are usually available in hospitals for lumbar puncture procedures. A complete kit would include the following:

1. Skin preparation materials, including sterile sponges, povidone-iodine swabs, and alcohol swabs
2. Sterile field, including sterile towels and drapes
3. Sterile gloves
4. Mask
5. Local anesthetic, usually lidocaine 1% plain
6. Syringe (3 ml) and needles (22 gauge × 1½ inch, 25 gauge × ⅝ inch)
7. Spinal needles (both 18 and 20 gauge, 3-inch length)
8. Three-way stopcock
9. Sterile collection tubes
10. Manometer
11. Gauze dressings and adhesive bandage

■ ANATOMY/APPROACH

Anatomy

Important spinal anatomy is reviewed in Figure 28–1. The spinal cord proper ends at L1-2 and continues as the cauda

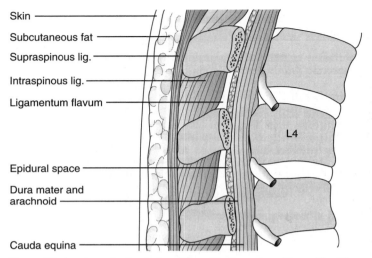

Skin
Subcutaneous fat
Supraspinous lig.
Intraspinous lig.
Ligamentum flavum

L4

Epidural space
Dura mater and
arachnoid

Cauda equina

Figure 28–1 □ Important spinal anatomy. (Redrawn from Brown DL: Atlas of Regional Anesthesia. Philadelphia, WB Saunders Co, 1999, p. 317.)

equina. Note the interspinous ligament and the ligamentum flavum, each of which is traversed when a needle is passed between two vertebrae. Figure 28–2 shows the advancement of a needle through the skin between L3 and L4, penetration of the subcutaneous tissue and interspinous ligament, and entry into the subarachnoid space containing the cauda equina.

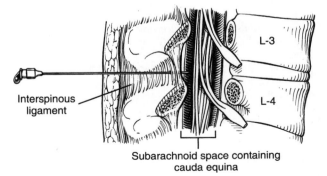

L-3

L-4

Interspinous
ligament

Subarachnoid space containing
cauda equina

Figure 28–2 □ Penetrating tissue layers to enter the subarachnoid space. (From Brown DL: Regional Anesthesia and Analgesia. Philadelphia, WB Saunders Co, 1996, p. 331, by permission of Mayo Foundation.)

Approach

There are two approaches to a spinal tap.

Lateral Decubitus Approach

The lateral decubitus approach (Fig. 28–3) is the favored approach for most patients. The patient should lie in the lateral decubitus position at the edge of the bed, with the knees, hips, and back maximally flexed. The knees should rest near the chest. The more flexed the patient, the more space is opened between L3 and L4 for passage of the needle. The shoulders and hips of the patient should be perpendicular to the bed.

Sitting Approach

For obese patients or patients with spinal disease or deformity, the sitting approach may be easier for both the physician and the patient. Ask the patient to sit at the edge of the bed. Have the patient lean over two pillows with his head flexed, as shown in Figure 28–4.

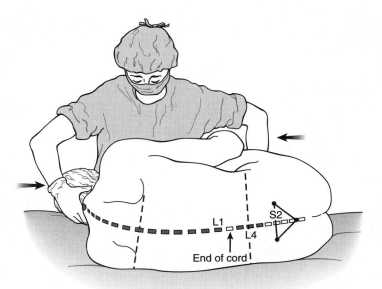

Figure 28–3 □ The lateral decubitus position for lumbar puncture. (Redrawn from Brown DL: Atlas of Regional Anesthesia. Philadelphia, WB Saunders Co, 1999, p. 316.)

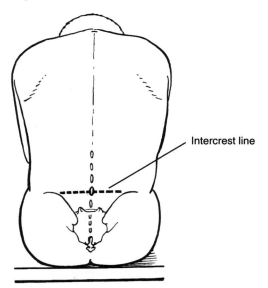

Intercrest line

Figure 28–4 □ Sitting approach for lumbar puncture. The intercrest line approximates L4. (From Brown DL: Regional Anesthesia and Analgesia. Philadelphia, WB Saunders Co, 1996, p. 330, by permission of Mayo Foundation.)

■ TECHNIQUE

1. Use sterile technique, and thoroughly prepare the middle and lower back with povodine-iodine solution.
2. Put on sterile gloves and a mask.
3. Palpate the midline.
4. Identify the L4–5 space. (Recall that L4 lies at the level of the iliac crests.)
5. Infiltrate the skin with local anesthetic agent with the 25-gauge needle. Replace the 25-gauge needle with the 22-gauge needle, and advance the local anesthetic agent into the interspinous tissues to provide deeper analgesia.
6. Insert the spinal needle into the skin.
7. Using two hands to guide the needle, slowly advance the spinal needle with the stylet in. You may advance perpendicular to the skin or at most, at an angle of 10° cephalad (Fig. 28–5).
8. Use your fingertips to feel for a "pop" as the ligamentum flavum is perforated.
9. Withdraw the stylet and look for the drainage of CSF. Check to see how far the needle has been advanced. If the needle

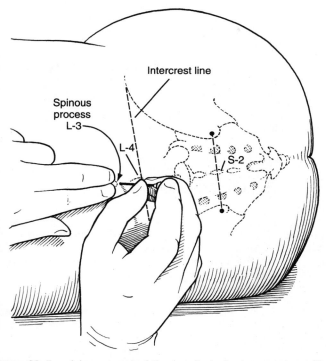

Figure 28–5 ▫ Advancement of the needle in lumbar puncture. (From Brown DL: Regional Anesthesia and Analgesia. Philadelphia, WB Saunders Co, 1996, p. 330, by permission of Mayo Foundation.)

has been advanced less than 4 cm, replace the stylet and slowly advance the needle in 2-mm increments. With each 2-mm advancement, remove the stylet and check for CSF drainage. If the needle has been advanced more than 4 cm in an adult, withdraw the needle and redirect.

10. Once CSF has been found, connect the needle to the three-way stopcock and attach the manometer (see Fig. 28–5).

11. Measure the opening pressure. Recall that normal opening pressures can vary from 70 to 180 mm CSF.

12. Collect the CSF, and obtain separate samples for the following:
    a. Cell count and differential
    b. Protein, glucose, and serology
    c. Gram stain, culture and sensitivity, acid-fast stain and culture, fungal stain and culture, and viral culture

13. Remove the needle.

14. Apply the dressing.

15. Instruct the patient to remain supine in bed for at least 12 hours to minimize the risk of headache and other complications.

■ COMPLICATIONS/PROBLEMS

1. Brain herniation
   This disastrous complication can occur if a spinal tap is performed in a patient with increased intracranial pressure with a mass present. If there is any sign of increased intracranial pressure, such as papilledema, a computed tomography scan should be performed to rule out any mass lesion before any spinal tap is performed.

2. Infection
   Meningitis or empyema can occur if contamination is introduced into the subarachnoid space or surrounding spaces. Absolute sterility must be maintained during the procedure. In addition, spinal tap should not be performed if there are infectious processes near the lumbar puncture site; this includes skin lesions, subcutaneous masses, and spinal infections.

3. Subdural hematoma
   This can occur if a large volume of CSF is withdrawn rapidly from an elderly or a fragile patient. Perforating veins may tear and bleed into the subdural space.

4. Bloody tap or spinal epidural hematoma
   Bloody taps occur when anterior or lateral venous plexus vessels are lacerated by an excessively lateral or deep needle penetration. These are usually benign and self-limited bleeds.

5. Headache

This is a common complication of lumbar puncture, occurring in as many as 25% of procedures. It is caused by the continued drainage of CSF into tissues outside of the subarachnoid space. Most common in young patients, the headache can last as long as 1 week after the lumbar puncture. Treatment includes strict bedrest, adequate hydration, and analgesia. Gross drainage of CSF through the skin puncture site requires consultation with a neurosurgeon for consideration of a blood patch.

THORACIC PROCEDURES

□ □ □

□ **29** □

TUBE THORACOSTOMY

Percutaneous drainage of the pleural cavity may be diagnostic and therapeutic. In the setting of dyspnea and hypoxia, the need for a chest tube is an emergent event. In the stable patient, take the extra time necessary to adequately prepare and sedate the patient.

Placement of Tube Thoracostomy

■ INDICATIONS

1. Pneumothorax
2. Pyothorax
3. Hemothorax
4. Chylothorax
5. Persistent pleural effusion

■ PRECAUTIONS

1. Coagulopathy
   Abnormalities in platelet count or function or in clotting factor concentrations should be corrected before insertion of the line.
2. Skin infection over the site of needle insertion may carry infection into the pleural cavity.
   Try to choose an uninvolved site.

■ EQUIPMENT NEEDED

1. Skin preparation supplies (iodine, chlorhexidine, or alcohol)
2. Local anesthetic (1% or 2% lidocaine, 25-gauge needle, 3-ml syringe)
3. Sterile gloves
4. Sterile towels or drapes

5. Sedative medication as necessary
6. Pulse oximeter
7. Chest tube of the appropriate diameter: thin for air removal, and thicker for fluid removal
   The perforated end may be cut down to facilitate a smaller patient. Placing a bevel on the end is not recommended; it may facilitate placement, but it is a perforation risk once inside the patient.
8. A chest tube insertion tray that includes blades, gauze, hemostats, trocars, thick silk suture with needle, and drapes
9. Petroleum gauze
10. Wide, gas-impermeable, occlusive tape
11. Suction device (i.e., wall suction)
12. Chest tube suction apparatus (Pleur-Evac) prefilled with water and hooked to the suction device

■ ANATOMY/APPROACH

The size and placement of the tube depend on the indication. A larger tube (36–40 Fr) and posterior placement are indicated for drainage of fluid; a smaller tube (24–28 Fr) and anterior placement are necessary for the drainage of air. The most versatile approach is laterally at the sixth interspace midaxillary line, about the level of the nipples. From this site, the tube may be directed either anteriorly or posteriorly.

■ ANESTHESIA

Local, with optional IV sedation and narcotic pain medicine. Conscious sedation is recommended for elective tube placement. (See Chapter 4.)

■ TECHNIQUE (STERILE)

Elective chest tube placement in a relatively stable patient may be done in a controlled and safe manner using adequate premedication of the patient with sedatives and local anesthesia. This technique describes a hemostat technique; some prefer a trocar-assisted placement. In an unstable patient, defer to the most experienced hands, do not take the time necessary to premedicate, and move as quickly and safely as possible.

1. **Prepare the patient.**
   a. Explain the procedure.
   b. Explain the risks and alternatives.
   c. Answer any questions.
   d. Have a consent form prepared and signed.

2. **Position of the patient.**

   Supine with the arm on the affected side extended upward

3. **Premedicate the patient.**

   a. Short-acting benzodiazepine such as lorazepam (Ativan) 1 to 5 mg IV.

   b. Short-acting narcotic such as fentanyl (Sublimaze) 25 to 50 μg IV also may be necessary.

   c. Skip all premedication (both benzodiazepine and narcotic) if the patient is dyspneic or is at risk for respiratory depression.

4. **Prepare the skin.**

   a. Use sterile technique and sterile gloves, mask, and gown.

   b. Plan the incision.

      The midaxillary line is generally used, with anterior direction of the chest tube to remove gas and posterior direction of the chest tube to remove fluid. Plan to make the skin incision about 2 to 3 cm below the rib interspace to be entered so that there is an oblique skin channel. This usually facilitates skin closure on removal of the tube. On occasion, the anterior midclavicular line is used to treat uncomplicated pneumothorax.

   c. Sterilely prep and drape the skin.

   d. Infiltrate with 1% to 2% lidocaine into the skin at the entry site and over the rib at the selected interspace.

      The periosteum of the top of the rib is very sensitive; do not skimp on lidocaine. Infiltrate the subcutaneous tunnel as well while removing the needle.

5. **Make the skin incision over a rib** (Fig. 29–1).

   Confirm adequate anesthesia. Cutting over the bone allows a clean, deep cut and avoids the neurovascular bundle that travels the underside of each rib. The incision should be about 1.5 times the diameter of the chest tube. Control any bleeding with pressure. Reinject with lidocaine as necessary (see Fig. 29–1A).

6. **Place a purse-string suture at the skin entry site.**

   Position the tie such that the loose ends are positioned inferiorly to the tube exit site, and place a single throw loosely.

7. **Bluntly dissect toward the pleura** (see Fig. 29–1B).

   a. Using a hemostat, create a subcutaneous channel superiorly from the skin incision to over the top of the rib at the desired interspace.

   b. Spread the hemostat to ensure that there is sufficient room for the diameter of the chest tube.

   c. Using a fair amount of pressure and with the hemostats closed, force the hemostats between the ribs through the intercostal muscles. **Stay right on top of a rib to avoid the neurovascular bundle.**

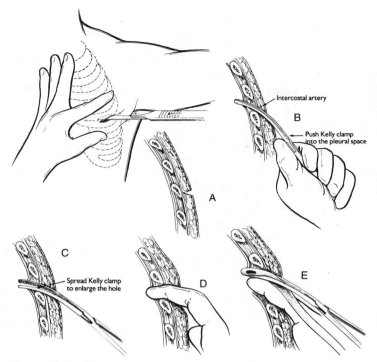

Figure 29–1 □ Thoracostomy tube placement. (From Dunmire SM, Paris PM: Atlas of Emergency Procedures. Philadelphia, WB Saunders Co, 1995.)

    d. You will notice a "pop" when the pleural cavity has been entered. Often, there also is a noticeable gush of air or fluid through the wound.

    e. Spread the hemostat tips to create sufficient space in the intercostal muscles to allow the tube to pass (see Fig. 29–1C).

    f. Remove the hemostat and insert a finger to confirm penetration into the pleural cavity (see Fig. 29–1D).

8. Insert the chest tube (see Fig. 29–1E).

    Using the hemostat, grasp the perforated end of the chest tube and place the tube through the subcutaneous channel and the intercostal muscle opening. This often is a difficult maneuver; it may take several passes to find the channel you created. (With trocar insertion, the tube is placed over the trochar and forced into the pleural cavity without hemostat perforation of the intercostal muscles.)

9. **Position the chest tube.**

Note that the chest tube has a mark just beyond the last perforations. When the tube has been placed into the chest and directed in the appropriate direction, insert the tube to the desired length. Make sure the mark is either inside the chest wall or just visible at the skin incision line, or the tube will leak.

10. **Secure the tube.**

Pull the purse-string suture snugly around the tube without adding throws. Wrap the loose ends around the tube several times to hold it in place. Make sure that several inches of suture are wrapped around the tube because this will be used to close the wound when the tube is removed. Once wrapped, the loose ends may be tied down securely (Fig. 29–2).

11. **Connect the chest tube to the Pleur-Evac and to wall suction.**

The suction pressure is defined by the volume of water (in cm of H_2O) in the suction control chamber of the Pleur-Evac. Bubbling in the underwater seal chamber will indicate adequate suction to remove gas and will continue for as long as there is an air leak. If fluid is to be removed, it will collect in the collection chamber (Fig. 29–3).

12. **Tape the chest tube site.**
    a. Wrap the tubing at the skin site with petroleum gauze.
    b. Apply occlusive tape in such a way that the tube site is relatively airtight and the tube is safe from being dislodged.

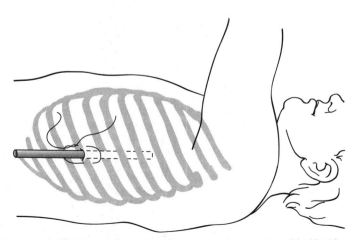

Figure 29–2 □ Purse-string ligature around chest tube site. (Modified from Adams GA, Bresnick SD: On Call Surgery. Philadelphia, WB Saunders Co, 1997, p 358.)

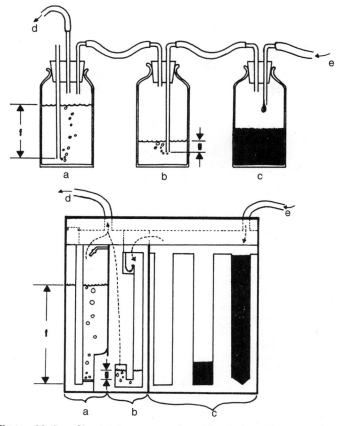

Figure 29–3 □ Chest tube apparatus. *a,* Suction control chamber. *b,* Underwater seal. *c,* Collection chamber. *d,* To suction. *e,* From patient. *f,* Height equals amount of suction in units of cm H_2O. *g,* Height equals underwater seal in units of cm H_2O. (From Marshall SA, Ruedy J: On Call Principles and Protocols, 2nd ed. Philadelphia, WB Saunders Co, 1993, p 180.)

    c. Further secure the tube by applying an "umbilical" tape such that unexpected pulls on the tube will pull on the umbilicus instead of on the suture (Fig. 29–4).

13. **Confirm tube placement by stat bedside upright AP chest x-ray (CXR).**

    Reposition as necessary. Daily CXRs are recommended to follow the course of therapy and to confirm continued ade-

Chest tube

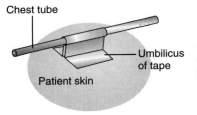

Umbilicus of tape

Patient skin

Figure 29–4 □ Tape umbilicus technique for securing chest tubes. (From Adams GA, Bresnick SD: On Call Surgery. Philadelphia, WB Saunders Co, 1997, p 360.)

quate placement of the tube. A lateral CXR may be helpful to find the exact location of the tube.

The most proximal hole in the chest tube interrupts the radio-opaque band on the tube, so it is easy to determine on CXR whether the tube is adequately placed. This most proximal hole should be well within the pleural space.

14. **Control the patient's pain.**

   The tube insertion site will remain uncomfortable until the tube is removed, so make sure the patient has adequate pain relief.

15. **Pulmonary toilet is important in a patient with a chest tube.**

   Make an incentive spirometer available, and instruct the patient as to its use and importance.

16. **Send fluid efflux from the chest tube to the laboratory.**

   The following studies may be indicated:
   a. Gram stain.
   b. Cultures (aerobic and anaerobic bacterial, fungal, mycoplasmal)
   c. TB culture and acid-fast bacilli (AFB)
   d. Cell count and differential
   e. LDH
   f. Protein
   g. Glucose
   h. Cytology for malignant cells
   i. Other studies as appropriate (amylase, triglycerides, pH, rheumatoid factor, antinuclear antibodies or complement levels, and so on)

   Blood for simultaneous tests for serum LDH, protein, glucose, and so on should be drawn to compare with the results of the pleural fluid.

17. **Document the procedure.**

■ COMPLICATIONS/PROBLEMS

1. Lack of resolution of the problem

   Occasionally, more than one chest tube will be needed.

2. Perforation of the lung
   This is more likely with a trocar placement.
3. Perforation of abdominal viscera
   This may happen if the skin entry site is too far caudal on the chest wall.
4. Perforation of the heart
5. Persistent air leak
   a. Check the tubing between the drainage apparatus and the patient for loose connections.
   b. Untape the wound site and confirm that the chest tube is inserted properly.
      Check whether the chest tube is fully inserted and the line is at or inside the skin line.
   c. If the entry site is not well closed, or a "sucking" sound is noted at the site, it may be necessary to further close the site with 2-0 silk sutures.
      Be sure to adequately prep and anesthetize the area before repair.
   d. Reposition the chest tube if necessary, and redress the site using petroleum gauze.
   e. If the connections are intact and the site is dressed in an airtight manner, order a portable AP CXR to assess the patient's lungs and the tube position.
   f. If the CXR shows lack of resolution of pneumothorax, consider placement of a second tube.
6. Persistent fluid efflux
7. Bleeding at the entry site
8. Discomfort

Pleurodesis Through a Tube Thoracostomy

In settings of persistent pneumothorax or malignant effusion, it may be necessary to perform pleurodesis. This entails infusion of an irritant into the pleural space to create scarring between the visceral pleura and the parietal pleura. On removal of the tube, the lung will remained scarred to the chest wall. Table 29–1 shows the agents typically used for pleurodesis.

■ INDICATIONS

1. Persistent malignant effusion
2. Persistent pneumothorax

Table 29–1 □ **AGENTS USED IN PLEURODESIS**

Agent	Concentration
Talc	2 g/100 ml NS
Tetracycline	1 g/100 ml NS
Doxycycline	1 g/100 ml NS
Bleomycin	60 IU/100 ml NS

■ CONTRAINDICATIONS

Hypersensitivity to lidocaine or the sclerosing agents

■ EQUIPMENT NEEDED

1. Tube preparation supplies (iodine, chlorhexidine, or alcohol)
2. 40 ml 1% lidocaine
3. Sterile gloves
4. Sedative medication as necessary
5. Pulse oximeter
6. 60-ml syringes (2) with 18-gauge needles attached
7. Tubing clamps (2)
8. Pleur-Evac
9. Sclerosing agent as prepared above (see Table 29–1)

■ ANESTHESIA

Premedication of the patient with both a narcotic and an anxiolytic medication.

■ TECHNIQUE (STERILE)

1. **Prepare the patient.**
   a. Explain the procedure.
   b. Explain the risks and alternatives.
   c. Answer any questions.
   d. Obtain informed consent if necessary.
   e. Place the patient on continuous pulse oximetry.
2. **Position of the patient.**
   Supine
3. **Premedicate the patient.**
   a. Short-acting benzodiazepine such as midazolam (Versed) 1 to 5 mg IV or lorazepam (Ativan) 1 to 5 mg IV.
   b. Short-acting narcotic medication, such as fentanyl (Sublimaze) 25 to 50 μg IV, also may be necessary.

4. **Prepare the tube.**
   a. Clamp the chest tube on the soft rubber portion close to the patient.
   b. Sterilely prepare a portion of the rubber tubing proximal to the clamp.
5. **Inject 40 ml 1% lidocaine into the tube.**
6. **Elevate the tube so that the entire volume enters the chest cavity.**
7. **Place a second clamp on the tube on the plastic portion just at the chest wall.**
8. **Position the patient as follows:**
   a. 2 minutes supine Trendelenburg
   b. 2 minutes supine reverse Trendelenburg
   c. 2 minutes right lateral decubitus
   d. 2 minutes left lateral decubitus
   e. 2 minutes prone (optional)
9. **Unclamp the tube at the site closest to the patient and inject the sclerosing agent into the tube.**
10. **Elevate the tube so that the entire volume enters the chest cavity.**
11. **Reclamp the tube on the plastic portion just at the chest wall.**
12. **Position the patient as follows:**
    a. 15 minutes supine Trendelenburg
    b. 15 minutes supine reverse Trendelenburg
    c. 15 minutes right lateral decubitus
    d. 15 minutes left lateral decubitus
    e. 15 minutes prone (optional)
13. **Unclamp the tube and allow the sclerosing agent to drain.**
14. **Reconnect the chest tube to suction for 24 to 48 hours or until there is no persistent air leak.**
15. **Document the procedure.**

■ COMPLICATIONS

1. If the patient becomes dyspneic or hypoxic at any time during the procedure, unclamp the chest tube and return it to suction.
2. Incomplete pleurodesis is common. If there are persistent symptoms, repeat application of pleurodesis or a surgical decortication may be necessary.

Removal of Tube Thoracostomy

This is best done with an assistant.

1. Confirm that the patient is ready to have the chest tube removed.
   a. There should be no persistent air leak, or the patient

should have been stable for at least 24 hours on water
seal alone.
  b. Ongoing fluid leak or bleeding should have stopped.
  c. The lung should be inflated on CXR.
  d. There is no other reason to consider leaving the tube in
  place.
2. Have all equipment ready.
  a. Blade or scissors to cut the knot from the purse-string suture
  b. Petroleum gauze
  c. Wide, gas-impermeable occlusive tape
  d. Dry gauze sponges (4 in. × 4 in.)
  e. Pulse oximeter (as necessary)
  f. Gloves and eyewear
3. Explain the procedure.
     Removal of the chest tube will require patient cooperation,
  and it is somewhat painful. Explain well what is to occur.
  Use minimal administration of opiate pain medication because this may depress respiratory function.
4. Position the patient: upright or supine.
5. Remove existing tape.
6. Cut the purse-string suture at the knot, leaving the long ends
  intact, and unwrap from the chest tube.
7. Tighten the purse-string suture such that the skin closes
  tightly around the tube.
     Confirm that the tube is free from the suture and tape.
8. Remove the chest tube.
  a. Have the patient inhale completely and hold his or her
  breath at the peak of inhalation.
     This guarantees a positive pressure in the pleural cavity
  and does not leave room for an involuntary gasp by the
  patient when the tube is removed.
  b. While the patient is holding his or her breath, the first
  person pulls the chest tube out.
     The same individual should place the petroleum gauze
  over the skin site to avoid the influx of air.
  c. At the same time as the tube is being removed, the second
  person pulls the ends of the purse-string suture such that
  the skin seals tightly underneath the petroleum gauze bandage.
  d. Tie down the ends.
9. Apply dry gauze and occlusive tape to the site.
10. Obtain a CXR to assess for pneumothorax.
     A small amount of air is common and may be treated with
  100% O_2 therapy.
11. Observe the patient over the next few hours for adequate
  breath sounds and oxygenation.
12. Examine the patient in 24 hours and obtain a follow-up CXR.

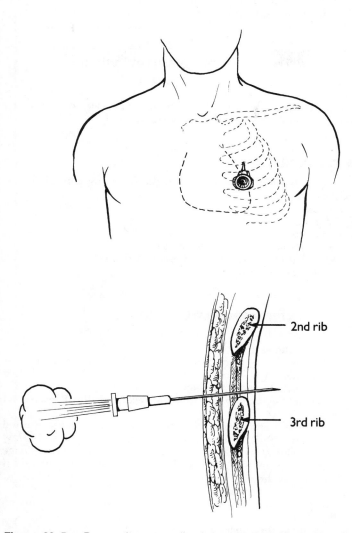

Figure 29–5 ▫ Pneumothorax needle decompression. (From Dunmire SM, Paris PM: Atlas of Emergency Procedures. Philadelphia, WB Saunders Co, 1995, p 56.)

If respiratory distress develops at any time, evaluate the patient for replacement of the chest tube.

Treatment of Emergent Tension Pneumothorax

Immediate action is required for decompression of acute tension pneumothorax. This is a **code** situation.

■ DIAGNOSIS

Suspect tension pneumothorax if the following clinical setting exists:
Hypoxia
Dyspnea
Hypotension
Hyperresonance on the affected side
Decreased breath sounds on the affected side
Jugular venous distention

■ TREATMENT (IMMEDIATE ACTION IS REQUIRED!)

1. **Prepare the skin.**
   If time allows, sterilely prepare the skin over the second or third intercostal space. Go two to three fingerbreadths below the clavicle to avoid the subclavian vessels.
2. **Insert a 16-gauge needle into the second or third intercostal space.**
   Approach anteriorly at the midclavicular line on the affected side (Fig. 29–5). This will confirm the diagnosis and allow some relief of symptoms until adequate chest tube drainage can be implemented. You should hear a gush of air outward if tension pneumothorax exists.
3. **Place a chest tube if needed.**
   If pneumothorax is confirmed, place a tube thoracostomy on the affected side.
4. **Document the procedure.**

30

THORACENTESIS

Thoracentesis is used to evacuate large volumes of fluid from the thoracic cavity for therapeutic or diagnostic benefit. Specific kits are available.

■ INDICATIONS

Diagnosis of pleural effusion, treatment of significant respiratory distress from pleural effusion, or both.

■ PRECAUTIONS

1. Coagulopathy
   Abnormalities in platelet count or function or in clotting factor concentrations should be corrected before insertion of the line.
2. Skin infection over the site of needle insertion may carry infection into the pleural cavity.
   Try to choose an uninvolved site.
3. Whenever a needle is inserted into the chest cavity, be prepared to place a tube thoracostomy (see Chapter 29).

■ EQUIPMENT NEEDED

1. Skin preparation supplies (iodine, chlorhexidine, or alcohol)
2. Local anesthetic (1% or 2% lidocaine, 25-gauge needle, 3-ml syringe)
3. Sterile gloves
4. Sterile towels or drapes
5. Pulse oximeter (as necessary)
6. A thoracentesis tray that includes drapes, syringes (one for specimens and a large one with a stopcock for large volume removal), sterile bottles for specimen collection, and a thoracentesis needle and catheter
7. Bottles for large volume collection
8. Sterile dressing supplies

■ ANATOMY/APPROACH

There is the danger of entering the abdominal cavity if the needle is inserted below the eighth interspace. In general, the effusion should be localized by percussion, and the needle should be inserted one to two fingerbreaths below the top of the effusion.

The patient should be sitting and leaning forward, as on the back of a chair (Fig. 30–1).

■ ANESTHESIA

Local

■ TECHNIQUE

Elective thoracentesis in a relatively stable and cooperative patient may be done in a controlled and safe manner under local anesthesia. Be sure to confirm the side to be tapped with a chest

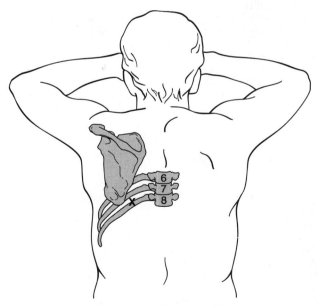

Figure 30–1 □ Patient position.

x-ray (CXR). It also may be useful to obtain a lateral decubitus film to see whether the fluid "layers out" in a dependent fashion. This suggests that the fluid will be accessible to drain.

1. **Prepare the patient.**
   a. Explain the procedure.
   b. Explain the risks and alternatives.
   c. Answer any questions.
   d. Have a consent form prepared and signed.
2. **Position of the patient.**
   Sitting, bent forward over the back of a chair
3. **Prepare the skin.**
   a. Plan the procedure. Percuss the back until lung dullness can be identified. Mark this level with pen on the patient's back. Plan to enter the skin at one to two interspaces below the top of the dullness; entering below the eighth interspace increases the risk of abdominal viscera perforation.
   b. Use sterile technique, and wear sterile gloves, mask, and gown.
   c. Sterilely prep and drape the skin over the affected side.
   d. Infiltrate with 1% to 2% lidocaine into the skin at the entry site and over the rib at the selected interspace. The periosteum of the top of the rib is very sensitive, so do not skimp on lidocaine.
4. **Insert the needle.**
   a. Most commercial kits use a catheter-over-needle approach.
   b. When adequate anesthesia has been achieved, insert the needle into the back, staying close to the top of the rib to avoid the neurovascular bundle, which travels the underside of each rib. It is safest to "march" up the rib with the needle to enter safely (Fig. 30–2).
   c. Aspirate frequently during needle advancement.
   d. You may feel a "pop" as the pleura is entered.
   e. A foreign body in the pleural space is very irritating, and the patient is likely to cough. Remind the patient of this before inserting the needle.
5. **Advance the catheter.**
   When fluid flows freely, advance the catheter over the needle into the pleural space. Aim down toward the posterior diaphragm.
6. **If no fluid flows**
   a. Confirm landmarks.
   b. Reinsert needle.
7. **Collect pleural fluid for diagnostic testing as follows:**
   a. Gram stain, cultures (aerobic and anaerobic bacterial, fungal, and mycoplasmal as indicated)
   b. TB culture and acid-fast bacilli (AFB)

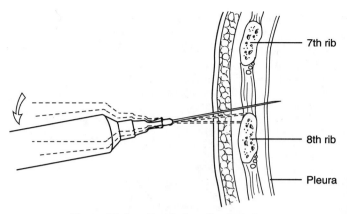

Figure 30–2 □ Needle insertion technique.

 c. Cell count and differential
 d. LDH
 e. Protein
 f. Glucose
 g. Cytology for malignant cells
 h. Other studies as appropriate (amylase, triglycerides, pH, rheumatoid factor, antinuclear antibodies or complement levels, and so on)

  Blood for simultaneous tests for serum LDH, protein, glucose, and so on should be drawn to compare with the results of the pleural fluid.

8. **Large-volume tap**

 If large-volume removal is required for therapy, change to the large syringe and hook up the collection bottles via the stopcock. Whenever the syringe is removed, place a gloved finger over the end of the catheter to avoid the undue inflow of air into the pleural cavity. Large suction bottles (500–1000 ml) may be used in lieu of a large syringe and stopcock if available.

9. **Do not remove more than 1500 ml at a time** to avoid reinflation pulmonary edema.

 A repeat tap may be performed in 24 hours if needed.

10. **Follow tap with a CXR to look for signs of pneumothorax.**

 Often, there will be great symptomatic relief without much radiographic change in the fluid level.

11. **Document the procedure.**

■ COMPLICATIONS/PROBLEMS

1. Lack of resolution of respiratory distress despite adequate fluid removal
   a. Support oxygenation and cardiac output.
   b. Confirm the diagnosis.
   c. Repeat the tap as deemed necessary.
2. Pneumothorax
3. Hemothorax
4. Empyema
5. Hemodynamic compromise if large volumes are removed

31

EMERGENCY PERICARDIOCENTESIS

If clinical suspicion for cardiac tamponade is high, diagnosis and treatment may be effected by pericardiocentesis. This is a **code** situation and should be done at the bedside only if the patient has hemodynamic collapse. Defer to the most experienced hands. Contact the ICU/CCU for assistance with the procedure.

■ INDICATIONS

1. Cardiac tamponade
2. Progressive pericardial effusion with hemodynamic compromise or impending shock

■ PRECAUTIONS

1. Coagulopathy
   Abnormalities in platelet count or function or in clotting factor concentrations should be corrected before insertion of the needle.
2. Skin infection over the site of needle insertion may carry infection into the pericardial sac.

■ EQUIPMENT NEEDED

1. Skin preparation supplies (iodine, chlorhexidine, or alcohol)
2. Local anesthetic (1% or 2% lidocaine, 25-gauge needle, 3-ml syringe)
3. Sterile gloves
4. Sterile towels or drapes
5. Pulse oximeter and electrocardiograph (ECG) monitoring
6. V lead for ECG
7. 16- to 18-gauge spinal needle
8. 20-ml syringe
9. No. 11 blade
10. Sample tubes

■ ANATOMY/APPROACH

The best approach is from the left paraxyphoid notch (Fig. 31–1).

■ ANESTHESIA

Local or none

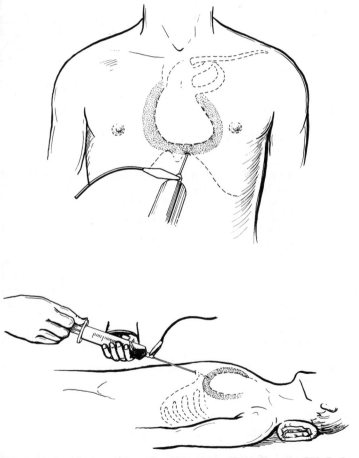

Figure 31–1 □ Approach to pericardiocentesis. (From Dunmire SM, Paris PM: Atlas of Emergency Procedures. Philadelphia, WB Saunders Co, 1995, p 64.)

■ TECHNIQUE (STERILE)

1. **Prepare the patient.**

   In an emergency situation, perform the procedure first when medically necessary.

   a. Explain the procedure.

   b. Explain the risks and alternatives.

   c. Answer any questions.

   d. Have a consent form prepared and signed.

2. **Position the patient.**

   The patient should be on continuous ECG monitoring and is best placed in a 30° semi-Fowler position if possible. Attach a V lead to the pericardiocentesis needle for greater sensitivity. An insulated wire with alligator clips at each end works well.

3. **Prepare the skin.**

   a. Use sterile technique, and wear sterile gloves, mask, and gown.

   b. Provide local skin preparation and draping over the xiphoid area.

   c. Perform local infiltration with 1% to 2% lidocaine into the skin at the entry site.

4. **Insert the needle.**

   a. Puncture the skin 2 cm below the costal margin to the left adjacent to the xiphoid with a blade (see Fig. 31–1).

   b. Direct the needle upward and posterior at a 45° angle for 4 to 5 cm.

   A good target at which to aim is the right or left scapular tip; the right is preferable because the risk of right ventricular penetration is lessened.

   c. Aspirate frequently as the needle is advanced.

   Continue to advance the needle until fluid is encountered, until cardiac pulsations are noticeable, or until ST elevation is noted on the ECG monitor. You may experience the sensation of entering a cavity.

5. **Remove blood if possible.**

   a. Most blood in a hemopericardium is clotted, so only 5 to 10 ml usually is removable.

   b. If 20 ml or more is easily withdrawn, then the needle most likely is in the right ventricle.

   c. A small aspiration of fluid often makes a big difference in cardiac function.

   d. If blood is encountered and is clotted or if no hemodynamic change is apparent after aspiration, the patient may need a thoracotomy or local pericardial window excision.

6. **Send fluid efflux to the laboratory.**

   The following studies may be indicated:

   a. Gram stain

   b. Culture (bacterial, fungal, and mycobacterial)

c. Hematological cell count
d. Cytology
e. Protein
f. Glucose
g. Other studies as indicated (rheumatoid factor, antinuclear antibodies, or complement levels)

7. **Document the procedure.**

■ COMPLICATIONS/PROBLEMS

1. Lack of resolution of the problem
   If persistent hemodynamic compromise is present despite adequate attempt at pericardiocentesis
   a. Reconfirm the diagnosis.
   b. Emergency thoracotomy or local pericardial window excision
2. Penetration of the myocardial wall
3. Myocardial infarction
4. Pneumothorax
5. Bowel perforation

URINARY DRAINAGE

□ □ □

32

TRANSURETHRAL
CATHETERIZATION

Many patients require urinary catheters for a variety of reasons. The on-call physician must understand how to place catheters in difficult situations when the nursing staff may be unable to catheterize or when the physician elects to catheterize the patient.

■ INDICATIONS

1. Urinary retention
2. Neurogenic bladder
3. Monitoring of urinary output
4. Retrograde irrigation of the bladder
5. Sterile urinary sampling

■ CONTRAINDICATIONS

1. Ureteral stricture: known and severe
2. Traumatic ureteral tears or lacerations
3. Acute infections of the urethra or prostate

■ PRECAUTIONS

1. Always use sterile technique.
   Meticulous attention to sterile technique is critical to avoid urinary tract infection. The placement of a urinary catheter introduces a foreign body to the urinary system, which greatly increases the risk of infection.
2. Always use a lubricant when placing a urinary catheter.
   This minimizes urethral trauma. Most urinary catheter kits come with a water-soluble lubricant.
3. Avoid traumatic catheter placement with multiple attempted passes.

If urethral narrowing or prostatic enlargement is suspected, quickly attempt smaller catheter or coudé catheter placement.

4. Be careful when placing urinary catheters in anticoagulated patients.

These patients tend to bleed easily. Use copious amounts of lubricants and nontraumatic technique.

5. Never inflate the Foley balloon without good urinary return and certainty of catheter placement in the urinary bladder.

Inflation of a Foley balloon in the urethra will likely traumatically tear the urethera.

■ EQUIPMENT NEEDED

1. Catheterization kit
   a. Skin preparation supplies (povidone-iodine solution)
   b. Sterile gloves
   c. Sterile gauze sponges
   d. Sterile towels
   e. Urinary catheter, usually Foley No. 16 or 18
   f. Water-soluble lubricant
   g. Syringe (10 ml)
   h. Sterile water or saline (5 ml)
   i. Adhesive tape
   j. Urinary drainage system
      1. Tubing
      2. Bag
   k. Optional items
      1. Lidocaine 2% jelly
      2. Coudé catheter
2. Urinary catheters

There are a variety of urinary catheters available (Fig. 32–1). The Foley catheter (see Fig. 32–1A) has a double-lumen shaft. The larger lumen allows urinary drainage, whereas the smaller lumen allows inflation of a 5-ml balloon, which anchors the catheter in the bladder. Foley catheters are the first-line drainage catheters used for transurethral drainage.

Figure 32–1B shows a straight catheter (red Robinson catheter). This type is most commonly used for straight, or "in-and-out," catheterization.

Figure 32–1C demonstrates a coudé catheter, which is used in difficult catheterizations. The tip of this catheter is narrowed and curved and is firmer than Foley catheters. This design allows the coudé catheter to pass through urethral narrowings or prostatic enlargements that inpinge on urethral patency.

Figure 32–1D shows a three-way irrigation catheter, which is used to retrogradely irrigate the bladder after urologic surgery.

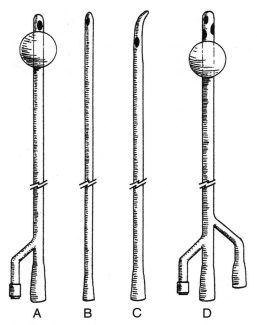

A   **B**   **C**   **D**

Figure 32–1 □ Urethral catheters. *A,* Foley catheter. *B,* Straight (red Robinson) catheter. *C,* Coudé catheter. *D,* Three-way irrigation catheter. For explanation, please see text. (From Marshall SA, Ruedy J: On Call: Principles and Protocols, 3rd ed. Philadelphia, WB Saunders Co, 2000.)

■ ANESTHESIA

1. No anesthesia is necessary for most patients.
2. Lidocaine 2% jelly can be used as both a lubricant and topical anesthetic agent. It can be injected into the urethra before catheter insertion.

■ TECHNIQUE

Male Patient

1. Position the patient supine.
2. Place sterile gloves and towels.
3. Retract the foreskin, if present.
4. Thoroughly prepare the entire penis, including the urethral meatus, with at least three passes of povidone-iodine solution.
5. Keep one hand sterile while the other holds the penile shaft.

6. Lift the penis straight upward as shown in Figure 32–2.
7. Lubricate the catheter tip and catheter shaft.
8. Insert the catheter into the urethral meatus.
9. Continue upward penile traction to straighten the urethra and ease catheter passage.
10. Advance the catheter slowly. Note the return of urine.
11. Only if urine drains, inflate the balloon with 5 ml of saline. If urine does not drain and the catheter is fully inserted, press on the bladder to start the flow of urine.
12. Gently pull back on the catheter until gentle resistance is appreciated.
13. Tape the catheter to the thigh with slight catheter slack, protecting the catheter from traction.

Female Patient

1. Position the patient supine.
2. Position the patient in frog-leg position or with knees spread.
3. Place sterile gloves and towels.
4. Expose the urethra using one hand by spreading the labia.
   Look for the vaginal orifice. The urethral meatus is anterior to the vagina and posterior to the clitoris. There is some

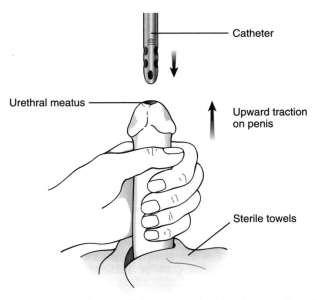

Catheter

Urethral meatus

Upward traction on penis

Sterile towels

Figure 32–2 □ Technique for Foley catheter insertion in the male patient.

minor variation in both appearance and location of the urethral meatus in female patients, so retraction of the labia and good visualization are critical to identify the urethra.

5. Lubricate the catheter tip and catheter shaft.
6. Insert the catheter into the urethral meatus.
7. Advance the catheter slowly; note the return of urine.
8. Only if urine drains, inflate the balloon with 5 ml of saline. If urine does not drain and the catheter is fully inserted, press on the bladder to start the flow of urine.
9. Gently pull back on the catheter until gentle resistance is appreciated.
10. Tape the catheter to the thigh with slight catheter slack, protecting the catheter from traction.

■ COMPLICATIONS/PROBLEMS

1. Difficulty passing the urinary catheter
   Causes: Meatal stricture, urethral stricture, prostatic enlargement, recent urologic surgery
   Solutions: A strictured meatus can be gently dilated with a curved hemostat; this may best be done by a urologist. Urethral stricture may be managed by the direct injection of sterile, water-soluble lubricant into the urethra and the passage of a coudé catheter. Care must be taken not to overtraumatize the urethra because edema may occur and further passage of catheters may become more difficult.
2. Transurethral tear and false passage
   Gentle technique must be used when placing urinary catheters. If the catheter is too small or too stiff and is placed with undue force, a urethral tear may occur. If this occurs, call a urologist.
3. Infection
   Contaminated catheter placement technique, contaminated catheters, preexisting infection, or other events can cause urinary tract infection or sepsis. Avoid infection through sterile catheter placement technique, good catheter care, appropriate catheter changes, antibiotic therapy as needed, and removal of urinary catheters as soon as they are no longer neccessary.
4. Traumatic placement resulting in hematuria
   Traumatic catheterization is the most common cause of hematuria. Urinary tract pathology or disease may also predispose to bleeding. The use of atraumatic technique is the key to avoiding injury to the urinary tract.

33

SUPRAPUBIC CATHETERIZATION

The placement of a suprapubic catheter is an important on-call procedure. When a urologist is not available and emergent bladder drainage is necessary, the on-call physician may be asked to place a suprapubic catheter. This is especially true in trauma cases. Care must be used in placing the catheter to avoid injuring abdominal and pelvic viscera.

■ INDICATIONS

1. Pelvic trauma causing urethral tear or disruption
2. Need for bladder drainage in the presence of urethral or prostate infection
3. Acute urinary retention when transurethral catheterization is not possible

■ CONTRAINDICATIONS

Nonpalpable bladder

■ PRECAUTIONS

1. Always use sterile technique.
   Meticulous attention to sterile technique is critical to avoid peritoneal or bladder infection. The placement of a suprapubic catheter introduces a foreign body into the bladder, which increases the risk of infection.
2. Avoid multiple needle passes when trying to cannulate the bladder.
   Each unsuccessful pass increases the risk of injuring the bowel or inducing bleeding.
3. Be careful when placing urinary catheters in anticoagulated patients.
   These patients tend to bleed easily; reversal of their anticoagulated status may be necessary to safely place a suprapubic tube.

■ EQUIPMENT NEEDED

1. Basic supplies
   a. Skin preparation supplies (povidone-iodine solution)
   b. Local anesthetic (1% lidocaine, with or without epinephrine; 22-gauge, 1½-inch needle 10-ml syringe)
   c. Razor
   d. Sterile gloves and mask
   e. Sterile gauze sponges
   f. Sterile towels and sheets
2. Cannulation equipment
   a. No. 11 scalpel
   b. Syringe (60 ml)
   c. Suprapubic catheter, usually 14-gauge, 12-inch
   d. Intracath needle
   e. Needle holder, scissors, and pickups
   f. Suture (2-0 silk or nylon)
   g. Adhesive tape
   h. Urinary drainage system
      1. Tubing
      2. Bag
   i. Sterile dressings
   j. Povidone-iodine ointment

■ ANATOMY/APPROACH

The urinary bladder is situated beneath the peritoneum (Fig. 33–1). When the bladder is empty, it is protected by the overlying

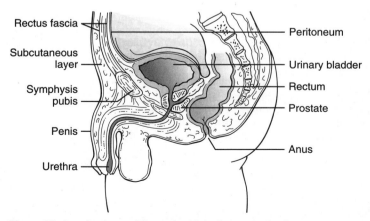

Figure 33–1 □ Anatomy of the male pelvis demonstrating important structures in relation to the urinary bladder.

symphysis pubis. The abdominal wall and rectus fascia lie superficial to the peritoneum, just below the skin and subcutaneous fat. For a needle to enter the urinary bladder, it must pass through these layers: skin, fat, rectus fascia, peritoneum, and bladder wall. It is critical that the bladder be distended so that it rises above the symphysis pubis and displaces loops of bowel. This minimizes the risk of bowel perforation with catheter placement.

■ ANESTHESIA

Local anesthetic agent with or without light sedation is appropriate for this procedure.

■ TECHNIQUE

This technique may be performed as a catheter-through-needle technique as described, or as a sterile Seldinger technique.

1. Position the patient supine (Figs. 33–2 to 33–4).
2. Place a roll under the hips to extend the abdomen and pelvis.
3. Palpate the bladder; it must be distended and palpable.
4. Shave the region from the umbilicus to the pubis.
5. Locate the site for puncture.

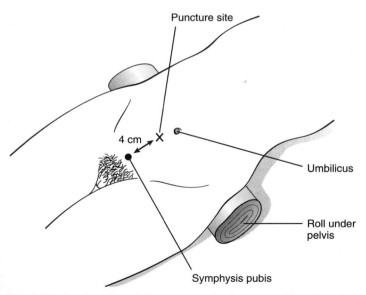

Figure 33–2 □ Location of the puncture site for suprapubic catheterization.

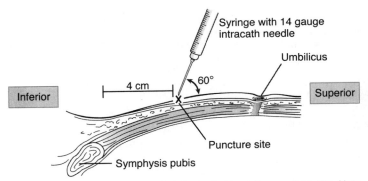

Figure 33–3 □ Cross section of abdominal skin at the puncture site. Note the angle between abdominal skin and the advancing needle.

The puncture site is in the midline, 4 cm above the pubis in an adult.

6. Clean the puncture site with alcohol solution.
7. Infiltrate a local anesthetic agent in the skin, subcutaneous layer, abdominal wall, and bladder wall. All layers to be penetrated should be anesthetized.
8. Thoroughly prepare the skin with povidone-iodine solution and drape with sterile towels and drapes.
9. Make a shallow skin incision in the puncture site with a No. 11 blade.
10. Using a 14-gauge Intracath needle on the 60-ml syringe, ad-

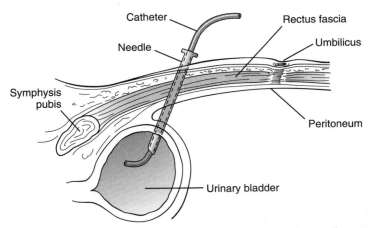

Figure 33–4 □ Threading the suprapubic catheter over the needle.

vance the needle through the incision at a 60° angle to the abdominal skin.

Advance the needle while aspirating until the needle tip is in the bladder and urine flows into the syringe.

11. Place the catheter in the bladder by removing the syringe from the needle and threading the Intracath catheter through the needle into the bladder. If the catheter returns urine, remove the needle over the catheter. Recheck that the catheter returns urine when aspirated. If urine flows freely, suture the catheter in place.
12. Attach a urinary collection device to the catheter.
13. Place a sterile dressing.

■ COMPLICATIONS/PROBLEMS

1. Difficulty passing the suprapubic catheter
   Cause: Needle tip not in urinary bladder lumen
   Solutions: Ensure that the needle freely aspirates urine and that the needle has not moved before threading the catheter.
2. Infection
   Causes: Contaminated catheter placement technique, contaminated catheters, preexisting infection, or other events can cause urinary tract infection or sepsis.
   Solutions: Avoid infection through sterile catheter placement technique, good catheter care, appropriate catheter changes, antibiotic therapy as needed, and removal of urinary catheters as soon as they are no longer neccessary.
3. Traumatic placement resulting in hematuria
   Causes: Traumatic catheterization is the most common cause of hematuria. A submucosal blood vessel in the bladder wall may be lacerated with the advancing needle. Urinary tract pathology or a rapidly decompressed bladder may also predispose to bleeding.
   Solutions: Small lacerated vessels generally stop bleeding spontaneously. If a bladder has been chronically distended, drain it slowly to decrease the risk of bladder lining tears and bleeding.
4. Bowel perforation
   Causes: If the needle is improperly positioned, inadvertent puncture of the bowel is possible. It is also critical that the bladder be distended before percutaneous bladder drainage. A distended bladder displaces bowel from the midline. If the bladder is not distended, the needle may first enter the bowel lumen.
   Solutions: Place a suprapubic tube only in a distended bladder. Avoid puncture more than 4 cm above the pubis. Always keep the puncture site in the midline.

LOCAL ANESTHESIA AND NERVE BLOCK

□ □ □

□ **34** □

LOCAL ANESTHESIA AND NERVE BLOCK

Local anesthesia, when properly administered, can provide profound pain relief and surgical anesthesia. Local anesthesia causes less disturbances of body physiology, prevents afferent impulses from the injury site from reaching the central nervous system, and can be easily administered in the on-call setting. Patients do not have to be nothing by mouth (NPO) before receiving a nerve block or infiltration anesthesia, and there are fewer complications than involved with general or regional anesthesia. This chapter reviews the important anatomy and techniques to allow the on-call physician to administer local anesthesia to the facial region and upper extremity with confidence.

■ INDICATIONS

1. Need for rapid analgesia or anesthesia
2. Patients at high risk for general or regional anesthesia (e.g., anticoagulated patients)
3. Limited region or block desired
4. Emergency procedures
5. Patients who have not been NPO
6. Limited injuries
7. Patients who would benefit from postprocedure analgesia
8. When no anesthesiologist or postprocedure monitoring is available
9. To provide anesthesia without loss or decrease in level of consciousness (e.g., patients with head injuries)
10. Patients with history of malignant hyperthermia

■ CONTRAINDICATIONS

1. Delay in onset of anesthesia
2. Complex surgical procedures

3. Procedures that may extend beyond the field of anesthesia
4. Long surgical procedures
5. When incomplete block is desired
6. Inexperienced practitioner
7. History of sensitivity to local anesthetic agents, requiring investigation (ester or amide anesthetics)
8. Patient refusal of local anesthetic agent
9. Patient inability to tolerate local anesthesia alone as an appropriate anesthetic (e.g., very young children, developmentally delayed persons)

■ PRECAUTIONS

1. Avoid the use of epinephrine distal to the wrist or ankle.

   In other words, do not use a local agent with epinephrine in the hand, foot, fingers, or toes. Generally speaking, it is not safe to use epinephrine in a cutaneous structure that is an "end organ." It *is* safe to use a local agent with epinephrine in the nose.
2. Avoid the use of epinephrine in the penis.
3. Avoid intravascular injection.

   Intravascular injection into a large vessel gives a rapid systemic absorption, which may lead to side effects such as cardiovascular depression or seizure. Always aspirate before injecting.
4. Always use aseptic technique.

   Do not infiltrate directly into a region of infection or spread contamination before the block. Always ensure that the skin is prepped with povidone-iodine solution or alcohol before the injection.
5. Consider the use of concurrent sedation if the procedure is more involved, a tourniquet outside the anesthetized area is used, or the patient is extremely apprehensive.
6. Provide appropriate preprocedure counseling and obtain consent.

■ EQUIPMENT NEEDED

1. Alcohol preparation or povidone-iodine
2. Sterile gloves
3. Local anesthetic agent; various options are available, and solutions may be mixed.
   a. Lidocaine options
      1. Lidocaine plain 0.5% or 1.0%
      2. Lidocaine with epinephrine 0.5% + 1:200,0000 or 1.0% + 1:100,000
   b. Bupivacaine (Marcaine) options
      1. Bupivacaine plain 0.25% or 0.5%

2. Bupivacaine with epinephrine 0.25% + 1:200,000 or 0.5% + 1:100,000
4. Short or long needle (25-gauge)
5. Syringe (3 to 5 ml)
6. Gauze, tape, and adhesive bandage

Field Block

■ ANATOMY/APPROACH

Field block, or infiltration block, refers to the placement of a local anesthetic agent into a region without making an effort to block a particular nerve. This is the easiest way to anesthetize the soft tissues in many areas of the body. This technique is commonly used in the face, upper extremity, trunk, and lower extremity. Even if there is a dominant nerve that innervates a particular area, the placement of a field block will often block afferent nerve fibers of the dominant nerve and provide the desired local anesthesia.

A field block works well to produce anesthesia in the skin and subcutaneous tissues. It is not generally effective for anesthetizing deeper structures, such as muscle or bone. Topical lidocaine can block muscle fascia, but muscle injuries and orthopedic injuries generally require major nerve block, regional block, intravenous analgesia, or general anesthesia to achieve adequate anesthesia.

In a field block, the local anesthetic agent diffuses to local nerve endings and nerve fibers and blocks the transmission of afferent impulses. Care should be taken to keep the agent just outside the region of injury, inflammation, or infection. Inflamed tissues are somewhat resistant to local anesthesia because of the acidic pH environment that surrounds inflamed tissue.

■ TECHNIQUE

1. Choose the local anesthetic agent.
   Consider your requirements regarding the duration of action. Always think about toxicity in choosing the local agent. Lidocaine is a good choice for durations of action that range from 30 to 90 minutes. Use lidocaine with epinephrine for longer duration of action within this range. If a longer duration is required or desired, bupivacaine with or without epinephrine offers a duration of action that ranges from 2 to 6 hours.
2. After skin preparation with alcohol or povidone-iodine solution, a ring of local anesthetic agent is injected into the subcutaneous tissue and intradermally.

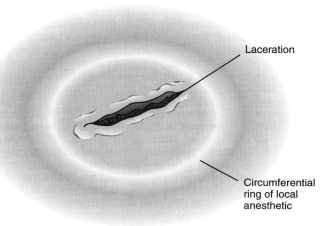

Figure 34–1 □ The concept of a field block. Local anesthetic is placed circumferentially around a wound or area to be anesthetized.

3. The local agent should be placed circumferentially around the injured region or the area to be anesthetized (Fig. 34–1).

Facial Nerve Block

■ ANATOMY/APPROACH

Although the most useful method to anesthetize a region of the face is a field block, there are instances when it is more useful to anesthetize an entire region of the face with one injection. This is often helpful in cases of facial trauma, in which large areas must be sutured. In other cases, tissue fragility after trauma makes it inappropriate to inject directly into injured tissue, and a facial block technique is useful. A common example seen in the emergency department is lip laceration that involves the vermillion border. Placement of the local anesthetic agent directly in the lip will distort the alignment of the lip with suture repair. However, the use of an infraorbital block or a mental block can anesthetize the lip without distorting it.

There are three major sensory nerves of the face; each is a terminal sensory branch of the trigeminal nerve. Figure 34–2 provides an overview of the many sensory nerves of the face,

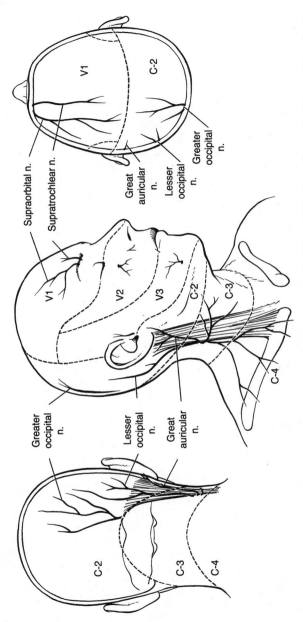

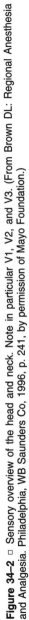

Figure 34–2 □ Sensory overview of the head and neck. Note in particular V1, V2, and V3. (From Brown DL: Regional Anesthesia and Analgesia. Philadelphia, WB Saunders Co, 1996, p. 241, by permission of Mayo Foundation.)

head, and neck. Pay close attention to the V1, V2, and V3 nerve distributions.

The Supraorbital Nerve

Figure 34–3 provides a close-up view of each major sensory branch of the trigeminal nerve. Note that the forehead is supplied by both the supraorbital nerve and the supratrochlear nerve. These nerves supply sensation to the entire forehead and parts of the upper eyelid. They exit from small bony foramen just at or above the superior orbital rim. The supraorbital nerve is usually found by palpating a notch in the superior orbital rim just vertically superior to the plane of the pupil of the eye.

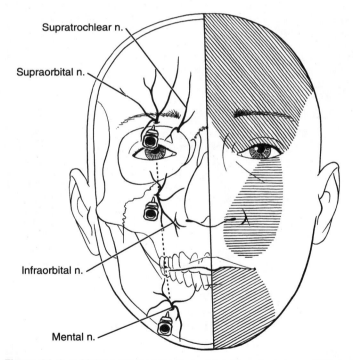

Figure 34–3 □ Major sensory branches of the trigeminal nerve (*left*) and areas of anesthesia achieved with nerve blocks (*right*). (From Brown DL: Regional Anesthesia and Analgesia. Philadelphia, WB Saunders Co, 1996, p. 244, by permission of Mayo Foundation.)

The Infraorbital Nerve

The midface, including the cheek and most of the upper lip, is supplied by the infraorbital nerve. This nerve exits from a bony foramen about 1 cm below the inferior orbital rim and 1 cm from the lateral side of the nose. This nerve is also vertically in line with the pupil. In infants and small children, care must be taken because the midface is short and the infraorbital nerve is generally closer to the orbit and eye. Infiltration block is generally safer in children and infants than infraorbital block, yet infraorbital block is extremely effective in adolescents and adults.

The Mental Nerve

The lower lip and chin are supplied by the mental nerve, which exits a bony foramen in the lower jaw. This nerve also lines up with the pupil of the eye about 1 cm above the lower mandibular border. The position of the foramen can be estimated by looking in the mouth and identifying the lower canine tooth and first molar on the side of interest. The foramen lies an equal distance between the canine tooth and first molar, about 1 cm from the lower bony edge of the mandible.

■ TECHNIQUE

1. The patient is placed supine in a relaxed position.
2. The anatomic region of the foramen is identified as described in the previous section.
3. The skin overlying the puncture site is prepared with alcohol.
4. The needle is inserted into the deep subcutaneous tissue layer, completely penetrating the skin, and 2 to 3 ml of local anesthetic agent is placed.
5. With supraorbital block, after the local agent is placed over the supraorbital foramen, the needle is partially withdrawn, redirected, and advanced 5 to 7 mm medially in the subcutaneous tissue layer, and an additional 1 to 2 ml of the local agent is placed. This anesthetizes the supratrochlear nerve.

Upper Extremity Block

The on-call physician is often asked to treat injuries to the forearm and hand; finger trauma is among the most common injuries seen on call. The regions of the upper extremity are best anesthetized by the on-call physician as follows:

1. Upper arm and forearm (infiltration block)

For anesthesia of the upper arm or forearm, infiltration block works extremely well. Local anesthetic, usually 3 to 5 ml with epinephrine, is injected into the superficial subcutaneous layer and dermis circumferentially around the injured area. In deeper injuries, the local agent can be safely injected with aspiration into deeper fascial layers and muscle. Up to 10 ml of a local agent can be used quite safely in the upper arm or forearm.

2. Hand and wrist (nerve block)

An understanding of the anatomy of the peripheral nerves at the wrist is critical to being able to provide local anesthesia with the nerve block technique. Figure 34–4 provides important anatomy of the wrist.

Nerve blocks at the wrist have many advantages for hand or finger injuries compared with other forms of anesthesia. The local agent can be administered proximal to the injury and in an uncontaminated field. The zone of anesthesia is large,

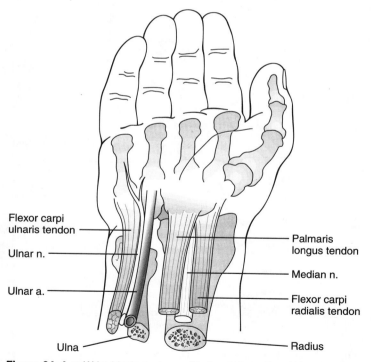

Figure 34–4 □ Wrist block anatomy. (Redrawn from Brown DL: Atlas of Regional Anesthesia. Philadelphia, WB Saunders Co, 1999, p. 62.)

blocking the entire distribution of the peripheral nerve of interest.

3. Finger (digital block) This simple technique requires injection of 1 to 2 ml of local anesthetic *without* epinephrine into the desired finger to achieve a dense finger block.

■ ANATOMY/APPROACH

The ulnar nerve lies on the ulnar (medial) side of the hand, just lateral to the flexor carpi ulnaris tendon (Fig. 34–5). This

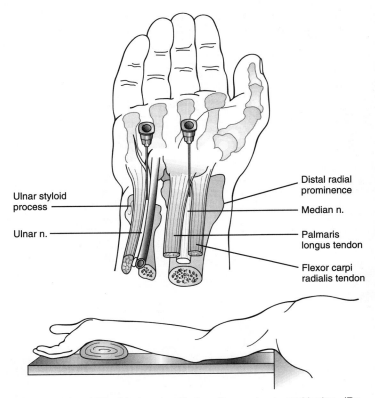

Figure 34–5 □ Wrist blocks—needle insertion and arm positioning. (Redrawn from Brown DL: Atlas of Regional Anesthesia. Philadelphia, WB Saunders Co, 1999, p. 63.)

tendon is easily palpable as the most medial wrist tendon at the ulnar border of the wrist. The ulnar nerve lies just medial to the ulnar artery.

The median nerve lies between the palmaris longus tendon and the flexor carpi radialis tendon. These two tendons are the most superficial tendons palpable on the inner side (volar) of the wrist. The palmaris longus tendon can easily be seen by asking the patient to oppose the thumb and little finger and to flex the wrist. The nerve is just deep to these tendons.

The radial nerve branches into multiple peripheral branches at the wrist level. These branches run in the subcutaneous layer in the dorsal and radial regions of the wrist. There is no distinct radial nerve trunk at the wrist level.

The digital nerves branch off main nerve trunks in the palm (see Fig. 34–5). Each finger has two main digital nerves that run down each side of the finger, primarily on the palmar side of each finger. There also are small dorsal nerve branches. The palmar digital nerves run with paired arteries. The palmar digital nerves supply sensation to the entire palmar side of the finger, including the fingertip and sides of the finger. The dorsal nerves run down the finger on the dorsal side and supply sensation to the dorsal skin and some of the nail bed.

■ TECHNIQUE

Ulnar Nerve Block

1. Position the patient supine with the arm extended (see Fig. 34–5). The wrist should be flexed over a small support such as a folded towel.
2. Palpate the flexor carpi ulnaris tendon. Palpate the pulse of the ulnar arter.
3. Prepare the region to be punctured with alcohol.
4. Insert a short 25-gauge needle between these structures, perpendicular to the skin of the wrist. In an adult, the nerve lies 5 mm below the skin surface.
5. Inject 3 to 5 ml of local *without* epinephrine after aspiration demonstrates that the needle is not in the ulnar artery or a vein.

Median Nerve Block

1. Position the patient supine with the arm extended (see Fig. 34–5). The wrist should be flexed over a small support such as a folded towel.
2. Identify the palmaris longus and flexor carpi radialis tendons in the central and radial wrist.
3. Prepare the region to be punctured with alcohol.

4. Advance a short 25-gauge needle between these two tendons and deep to them.
5. Inject 3 ml of local anesthetic agent *without* epinephrine after aspiration.

Radial Nerve Block

1. Position the patient supine with the arm extended (Fig. 34–6). The wrist should be flexed over a small support such as a folded towel.
2. Palpate the lateral edge of the radius bone (styloid process). The entire radial-dorsal region of the wrist, including the base of the anatomic snuff box, is visualized.
3. Prepare the region to be punctured with alcohol.
4. Advance a short 25-gauge needle into the subcutaneous tissue, and inject 5 to 6 ml of local anesthetic as a wide field block, extending from the radial-volar region, across the base of the anatomic snuff box, and ending in the dorsal-radial surface of the wrist.

Digital Nerve Block

1. Position the patient supine with the arm extended (Fig. 34–7). Ask the patient to position the hand with the palm down, fingers extended.
2. Prepare the base of the finger to be anesthetized with alcohol.
3. With a short 25-gauge needle (for adults), insert the local anesthetic agent on each side of the finger, at the finger base. The puncture site is lateral to the bone. The needle is inserted 7 to 10 mm for adults, with care taken to not perforate the

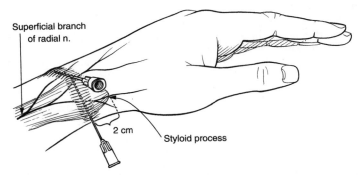

Superficial branch of radial n.

2 cm

Styloid process

Figure 34–6 □ The radial nerve block at the wrist. (From Brown DL: Regional Anesthesia and Analgesia. Philadelphia, WB Saunders Co, 1996, p. 274, by permission of Mayo Foundation.)

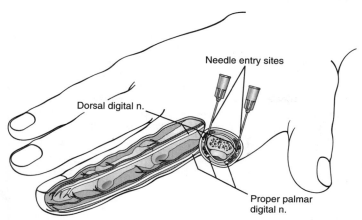

Figure 34–7 □ Digital block anatomy and needle insertion. (Redrawn from Brown DL: Atlas of Regional Anesthesia. Philadelphia, WB Saunders Co, 1999, p. 64.)

skin on the palmar side of the finger. No more than 1 ml of local anesthetic agent *without* epinephrine is injected.
4. If the dorsum of the finger is to be anesthetized, infiltrate 1 ml of local in the subcutaneous tissue of the dorsal skin of the finger, across the entire dorsal finger surface.

■ COMPLICATIONS/PROBLEMS

1. Poor analgesia
    This most often results from a poor understanding of the anatomy of the region to be anesthetized. When a block is missed, it usually means that the physician has placed the local agent in a poor location to anesthetize the nerve of interest. The physician may want to inject more local agent in a different tissue plane. Alternatively, other types of blocks can be used. If a nerve block is missed, one can use a field block instead. If a distal nerve block is missed (e.g., digital block), a more proximal nerve block (e.g., nerve block at wrist) can be used.
2. Allergic reaction to local anesthetic agent
    If a patient is allergic to the local agent that is used, treat the allergic reaction. Serious allergic reactions may require oxygen and subcutaneous epinephrine. Diphenhydramine (Benadryl) and systemic steroids may also be useful.
3. Systemic reaction to local anesthetic agent

The most serious side effects of local anesthetic agents include cardiovascular or neurologic reactions. If a local anesthetic agent is injected directly intravascularly or administered to a patient in an overdose, these reactions can occur. The reaction depends on the local given, whether it contained epinephrine, and the quantity given. Local without epinephrine can cause cardiac suppression. Local with epinephrine can cause overall cardiac stimulation owing to the epinephrine effect. Usually, little treatment other than monitoring is required.

ORTHOPAEDICS

□ □ □

SPLINTING

The on-call physician will often be asked to evaluate patients with sprains, ligamentous injuries, tendon injuries, or fractures. It is important to know how to stabilize the injured area so that the proper diagnostic and therapeutic treatments can be rendered. The application of an appropriate splint will comfort the patient and prevent further trauma or the displacement of a bony or soft tissue injury.

■ INDICATIONS

1. Bony fracture
2. Tendon laceration or avulsion
3. Joint injury or sprain
4. Extremity pain with movement

■ CONTRAINDICATIONS

None

■ PRECAUTIONS

1. Thin skin
   In patients with fragile skin, care must be taken to apply adequate padding under the splint. Several layers of cotton or web roll can be placed on top of the splint material to protect the skin. Failure to pad the skin can result in pressure sores and skin irritation.
2. Watch for swelling and avoid tight dressings.
   Swelling follows any significant soft tissue or bony injury. The advantage of a splint over a cast is that the splint allows for swelling as long as the wrap over the splint is relatively loose or contains gauze fluffs or cotton. It is important to give

the soft tissues room to swell in the first 24 to 48 hours following an injury.

3. Avoid moving injured parts until a radiographic or clinical diagnosis is reached.

The purpose of splinting is to protect an injured area until appropriate diagnostic or therapeutic care can be given. Do not attempt to manipulate an injured area when applying the splint. *Note:* It may be necessary to reduce some fractures into more anatomic position in order to regain impaired circulation or improve functional outcome.

■ EQUIPMENT

1. Plaster or fiberglass

   Both materials are acceptable, and each has advantages and disadvantages. Plaster is inexpensive and very rigid. The disadvantages of plaster are that it is heavy and prone to fracture. Fiberglass is lighter than plaster but quite expensive.

   Both plaster and fiberglass come as preprepared splinting material with foam padding embedded. If these "one-step" splints are not available in your hospital or clinic, you can make your own. Simply use 12 to 14 thicknesses of either plaster or fiberglass, and pad them with cotton or six to eight layers of web roll.

2. Cotton or web roll

   Web roll is a cotton-based material that comes in rolls of varying widths (3 to 6 inches).

3. Gauze fluffs

4. Bias roll or gauze rolls

5. Tape

6. Elastic wraps

7. Water

■ GENERAL TECHNIQUE

1. Select the splint material.

   a. Choose the appropriate width of splint to use.

      Three-inch splints work well for thumb splints, and 4-inch widths work well for wrist and elbow splints. Six-inch splints are useful for ankle, calf, and knee splints.

   b. Choose the splint thickness.

      If a prepackaged splint is used, there is no concern about thickness. If making your own splint, use at least 12 thickness for wrist splints and 15 thicknesses for elbow and lower extremity splints.

2. Ensure that the area is properly padded.
   a. For hand splints, place gauze fluffs between the fingers. Wrap the hand loosely with a gauze roll.
   b. Place at least 6 to 8 layers of web roll cotton padding beneath the splint to avoid pressure points.
   c. If a posterior splint is placed, ensure that at least 12 layers of cotton web roll cover the heel. The skin over the heel is prone to break down and form pressure sores.
3. Immerse the splint in water and wring out the excess water so that the splint is moist, not wet.
   Use cool water for fiberglass. Cool or warm water can be used for plaster. However, the warmer the water, the faster plaster sets.
4. Conform the splint to the area to be immobilized.
5. Wrap the splint with gauze rolls or bias rolls. Elastic wraps may be applied over gauze rolls to increase stability. Remember not to make elastic wraps too tight.

■ SPECIFIC TECHNIQUES

1. **Finger splinting**
   a. Simple finger fractures or sprains
      Finger fractures or sprains can be splinted by placing the finger in the fully extended position and immobilizing the finger with a volar splint. These splints are made of aluminum with foam padding (Fig. 35–1).
   b. Mallet finger deformity
      The mallet deformity involves rupture of the extensor tendon insertion onto the distal phalanx (Fig. 35–2A). This deformity may involve a fracture of the distal phalanx. If the distal phalax of a finger cannot be extended by the patient, this usually indicates extensor tendon injury, and

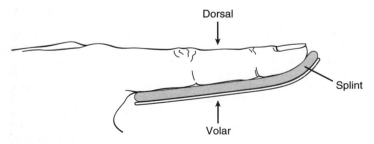

Figure 35–1 □ Aluminum splint with foam padding useful for volar splinting.

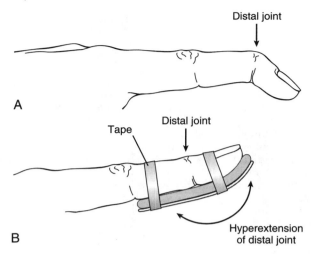

Distal joint

A

Tape   Distal joint

Hyperextension
of distal joint

B

Figure 35–2 □ *A*, The mallet deformity. The finger is fully extended and the dorsal joint does not extend. The finger looks like a "mallet." *B*, Splinting of a finger with a mallet deformity.

the finger should be splinted with an aluminum finger splint in a slightly hyperextended position, as shown in Figure 35–2*B*.

2. **Extensor tendon lacerations of the hands, wrists, or forearms**

These injuries should be splinted regardless of whether repair is performed at the same time. The goal of splinting these injuries is to take all tension off the injured tendon. The skin wound should be sutured and a protective dressing placed over the wound. Gauze fluffs should be placed between the fingers. The hand should be positioned with the wrist extended to 30°, the metacarpophalangeal joints should be flexed to 90°, and the proximal and distal interphalangeal joints should be in full extension. A protective splint should be fabricated to extend from the volar-proximal forearm to the volar fingertips (Fig. 35–3).

3. **Flexor tendon lacerations of the hands, wrists, or forearms**

Flexor tendon lacerations or avulsions must be splinted to prevent additional retraction of the lacerated tendon proximally. Appropriate splinting should take all tension off the injured tendon. The skin wound should be sutured and a protective dressing placed over the wound. Gauze fluffs should be placed between the fingers. The hand should be positioned with the wrist flexed to 30°, the metacarpophalangeal joints flexed to 45°, and the proximal and distal inter-

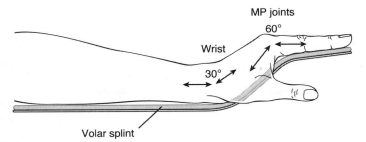

Figure 35–3 □ Wrist and metacarpophalangeal (MP) position in extensor tendon injuries. Formulation of a volar splint.

phalangeal joints flexed to 15° to 20°. A protective splint should be fabricated to extend from the dorsal-proximal forearm to the dorsal fingertips (Fig. 35–4).

4. **Injuries to the thumb: fractures, sprains, and tendon lacerations**

    The thumb is best protected with a thumb-spica splint. This splint is formulated with the thumb in 60° of abduction and fully extended (Fig. 35–5).

5. **Wrist sprains and fractures**

    Most wrist injuries are splinted in the wrist neutral position, with the wrist extended to 30°. A prefabricated wrist splint can also be placed for stabilization (Fig. 35–6).

6. **Elbow injuries**

    The elbow may be safely splinted with the elbow flexed between 45° and 90° with the palm facing up (supination). A

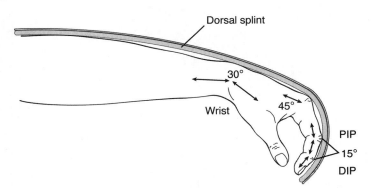

Figure 35–4 □ Wrist and finger joint position in flexor tendon injuries. Formulation of a dorsal splint.

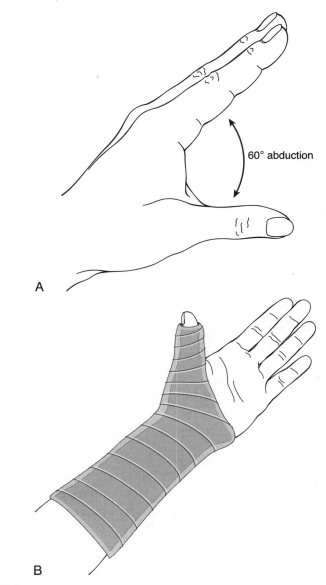

Figure 35–5 □ *A*, Abduction of the thumb for the placement of a thumb-spica splint. *B*, The thumb-spica splint for thumb immobilization.

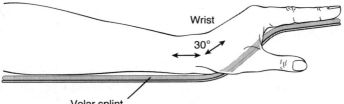

Figure 35–6 □ Volar splint for wrist sprains or fractures.

splint can be fabricated to sit on the posterior surface of the elbow area, extending from just below the shoulder to just proximal to the wrist (Fig. 35–7).

7. Ankle, Achilles tendon, and calf injuries

A posterior splint is the most appropriate immobilization for these acute injuries. Splint material is fabricated to extend

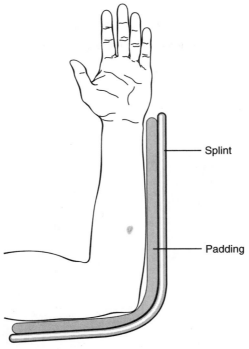

Figure 35–7 □ Elbow splint.

from the toes to just below the knee. Adequate padding must be used over the heel to prevent skin breakdown (Fig. 35–8).

8. Knee injuries

The knee is best splinted with a prefabricated knee immobilizer. These splints have internal metal struts for lateral knee support and Velcro straps to allow the immobilizer to be adjusted. This device holds the knee fully extended. No plaster or fiberglass splinting is required.

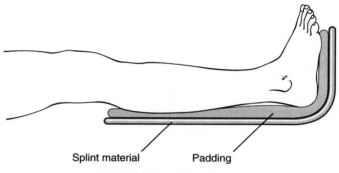

Splint material   Padding

Figure 35–8 □ Posterior splint.

APPENDICES

APPENDIX A

□ ⊡ □

READING X-RAYS, READING ECGs, ADULT EMERGENCY CARDIAC CARE ALGORITHMS

READING X-RAYS

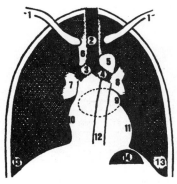

Figure A–1 □ Schematic of posteroanterior chest x-ray. (Reprinted from Marshall SA, Ruedy J: On Call Principles and Protocols, 3rd ed. Philadelphia, WB Saunders Co, 2000, p 417.)

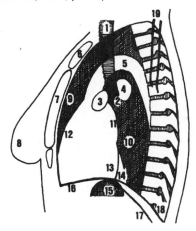

Figure A–2 □ Schematic of lateral chest x-ray. (Reprinted from Marshall SA, Ruedy J: On Call Principles and Protocols, 3rd ed. Philadelphia, WB Saunders Co, 2000, p 418.)

READING ECGs
Rate

Multiply the number of QRS complexes in a 6-second period (30 large squares) (between the two large dots) by 10 = beats/min (Fig. A–3).
- Normal = 60 to 100 beats/min
- Tachycardia = >100 beats/min
- Bradycardia = <60 beats/min

Rhythm

Is the rhythm regular?

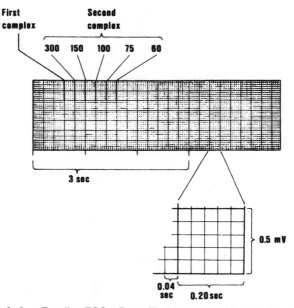

Figure A–3 □ Reading ECGs. Rate. (Reprinted from Marshall SA, Ruedy J: On Call Principles and Protocols, 3rd ed. Philadelphia, WB Saunders Co, 2000, p 405.)

Is there a P wave preceding every QRS complex? Is there a QRS complex following every P wave?
1. Yes = sinus rhythm
2. No P waves with irregular rhythm = atrial fibrillation
3. No P waves with regular rhythm = junctional rhythm. Look for retrograde P waves in all leads.

Axis

See Figure A–4.

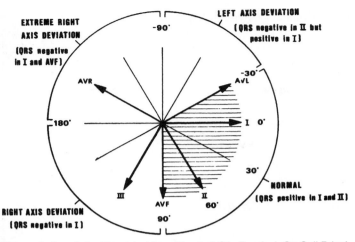

Figure A–4 □ Axis. (Reprinted from Marshall SA, Ruedy J: On Call Principles and Protocols, 3rd ed. Philadelphia, WB Saunders Co, 2000, p 406.)

P Wave Configuration

Normal P wave. Look at all leads (Fig. A–5*A*).

Left Atrial Enlargement (Fig. A–5*B*)

- Duration: 120 msec (three small squares in lead II). Often notched = P mitrale
- Amplitude: Negative terminal P wave in lead V_1 >1 mm in depth *and* >40 msec (one small square)

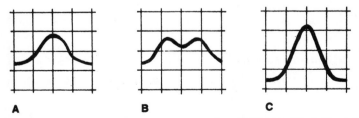

A   **B**   **C**

Figure A–5 □ Reading ECGs. P wave configuration in lead II. *A*, Normal P wave. *B*, Left atrial enlargement. *C*, Right atrial enlargement. (Reprinted from Marshall SA, Ruedy J: On Call Principles and Protocols, 3rd ed. Philadelphia, WB Saunders Co, 2000, p 406.)

Right Atrial Enlargement (Fig. A–5C)

- Amplitude: 2.5 mm in leads II, III, or aVF (i.e., tall, peaked P wave of P pulmonale); 1.5 mm in the initial positive deflection of the P wave in lead V_1 or V_2

QRS Configuration

Left Ventricular Hypertrophy

1. Increased QRS voltage (S in V_1 or V_2 plus R in V_5 >35 mm or R in aVL ≥11 mm)
2. Left atrial enlargement
3. ST-segment depression and negative T wave in left lateral leads

Right Ventricular Hypertrophy

1. R > S in V_1
2. Right-axis deviation (>+90°)
3. ST-segment depression and negative T wave in right precordial leads

Conduction Abnormalities

First-Degree Block

- PR interval ≥0.20 second (≥1 large square)

Second-Degree Block

Occasional absence of QRS and T after a P of sinus origin.
1. Type I (Wenckebach): Progressive prolongation of the PR interval before the missed QRS complex
2. Type II: Absence of progressive prolongation of the PR interval before the missed QRS complex

Third-Degree Block

Absence of any relationship between P waves of sinus origin and QRS complexes

Left Anterior Hemiblock

Left-axis deviation, Q in I and aVL; a small R in III, in the absence of left ventricular hypertrophy

Left Posterior Hemiblock

Right-axis deviation, a small R in I and a small Q in III, in the absence of right ventricular hypertrophy

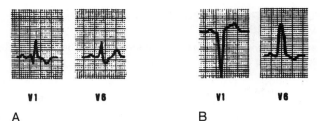

Figure A–6 □ Reading ECGs. QRS configuration. *A*, Complete right bundle branch block. *B*, Complete left bundle branch block. (Reprinted from Marshall SA, Ruedy J: On Call Principles and Protocols, 3rd ed. Philadelphia, WB Saunders Co, 2000, p 408.)

Complete Right Bundle Branch Block

See Figure A–6*A*.

Complete Left Bundle Branch Block

See Figure A–6*B*.

Ventricular Preexcitation

1. PR interval <0.11 second with widened QRS (>0.12 second) due to a delta wave = Wolff-Parkinson-White syndrome
2. PR interval <0.11 second with a normal QRS complex = Lown-Ganong-Levine syndrome

MYOCARDIAL INFARCTION PATTERNS

Type of Infarct	Patterns of Changes (Q Waves, ST Elevation or Depression, T Wave Inversion)*
Inferior	Q in II, III, aVF
Inferoposterior	Q in II, III, aVF, and V_6
	R > S and positive T in V_1
Anteroseptal	V_1 to V_4
Anterolateral to posterolateral	V_1 to V_5; Q in I, aVL, and V_6
Posterior	R > S in V_1, positive T, and Q in V_6

*A significant Q wave is >40 msec wide or > one third of the QRS height. ST-segment or T wave changes in the absence of significant Q waves may represent a non–Q wave infarct.

ADULT EMERGENCY CARDIAC CARE ALGORITHMS*

The Algorithm Approach to Emergency Cardiac Care

These guidelines use algorithms as an educational tool. They are an illustrative method to summarize information. Providers of emergency care should view algorithms as a summary and a memory aid. They provide a way to treat a broad range of patients. Algorithms, by nature, oversimplify. The effective teacher and care provider will use them wisely, not blindly. Some patients may require care not specified in the algorithms. When clinically appropriate, flexibility is accepted and encouraged. Many interventions and actions are listed as "considerations" to help providers think. These lists should not be considered endorsements or requirements or "standard of care" in a legal sense. Algorithms do not replace clinical understanding. Although the algorithms provide a good "cookbook," the patient always requires a "thinking cook."

The following clinical recommendations apply to all treatment algorithms:

- First, treat the patient, not the monitor.
- Algorithms for cardiac arrest presume that the condition under discussion continually persists, that the patient remains in cardiac arrest, and that CPR is always performed.
- Apply different interventions whenever appropriate indications exist.
- The flow diagrams present mostly class I (acceptable, definitely effective) recommendations. The footnotes present class IIa (acceptable, probably effective), class IIb (acceptable, possibly effective), and class III (not indicated, may be harmful) recommendations.
- Adequate airway, ventilation, oxygenation, chest compressions, and defibrillation are more important than administration of medications and take precedence over initiating an intravenous line or injecting pharmacologic agents.
- Several medications (epinephrine, lidocaine, and atropine) can be administered via the endotracheal tube, but clinicians must use an endotracheal dose 2 to 2.5 times the intravenous dose.
- With a few exceptions, intravenous medications should always be administered rapidly, in bolus method.
- After each intravenous medication, give a 20- to 30-ml bolus of intravenous fluid and immediately elevate the extremity. This will enhance delivery of drugs to the central circulation, which may take 1 to 2 minutes.
- Last, treat the patient, not the monitor.

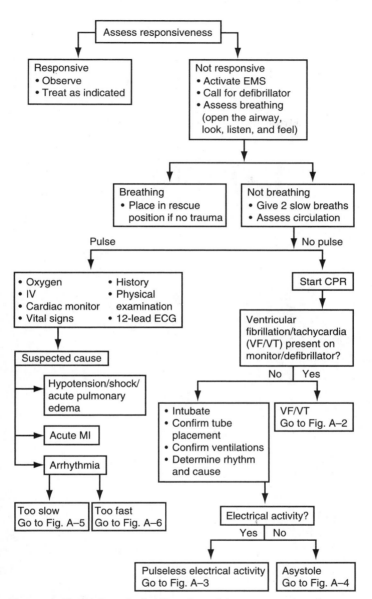

Figure A–7 □ Universal algorithm for adult emergency cardiac care (ECC). (Reproduced with permission from Journal of the American Medical Association: Guidelines for cardiopulmonary resuscitation and emergency cardiac care 1992, Vol. 268, CPR issue, pp 2199–2241, Copyrighted 1992, American Medical Association.)

Class I: definitely helpful
Class IIa: acceptable, probably helpful
Class IIb: acceptable, possibly helpful
Class III: not indicated, may be harmful

* Precordial thump is a class IIb action in witnessed arrest, no pulse, and no defibrillator immediately available.

† Hypothermic cardiac arrest is treated differently after this point. See section on hypothermia.

‡ The recommended dose of *epinephrine* is 1 mg IV push every 3–5 min. If this approach fails, several class IIb dosing regimens can be considered:
- Intermediate: *epinephrine* 2–5 mg IV push, every 3–5 min
- Escalating: *epinephrine* 1 mg–3 mg–5 mg IV push (3 min apart)
- High: *epinephrine* 0.1 mg/kg IV push, every 3–5 min

§ *Sodium bicarbonate* (1 mEq/kg) is class I if patient has known preexisting hyperkalemia.

‖ Multiple sequenced shocks (200 J, 200–300 J, 360 J) are acceptable here (class I), especially when medications are delayed.

¶ • *Lidocaine* 1.5 mg/kg IV push. Repeat in 3–5 min to total loading dose of 3 mg/kg; then use.
• *Bretylium* 5 mg/kg IV push. Repeat in 5 min at 10 mg/kg.
• *Magnesium sulfate* 1–2 g IV in torsades de pointes or suspected hypomagnesemic state or severe refractory VF
• *Procainamide* 30 mg/min in refractory VF (maximum total 17 mg/kg)

\# • *Sodium bicarbonate* (1 mEq/kg IV):
Class IIa
• If known preexisting bicarbonate-responsive acidosis
• If overdose with tricyclic antidepressants
• To alkalinize the urine in drug overdoses
Class IIb
• If intubated and continued long arrest interval
• On return of spontaneous circulation after long arrest interval
Class III
• Hypoxic lactic acidosis

Flowchart:

- ABCs
- Perform CPR until defibrillator attached*
- VF/VT present on defibrillator

↓

Defibrillate up to 3 times if needed for persistent VF/VT (200 J, 200–300 J, 360 J)

↓

Rhythm after the first 3 shocks?†

Branches:
- Return of spontaneous circulation
- PEA Go to Fig A–3
- Asystole Go to Fig A–4
- Persistent or recurrent VF/VT

Return of spontaneous circulation
• Assess vital signs
• Support airway
• Support breathing
• Provide medications appropriate for blood pressure, heart rate, and rhythm

Persistent or recurrent VF/VT
• Continue CPR
• Intubate at once
• Obtain IV access

↓

Epinephrine 1 mg IV push‡§ repeat every 3–5 min

↓

Defibrillate 360 J within 30–60 s ‖

↓

Administer medications of probable benefit (class IIa) in persistent or recurrent VF/VT¶#

↓

Defibrillate 360 J, 30–60 s after each dose of medication‖
Pattern should be drug-shock, drug-shock

Figure A–8 □ Algorithm for ventricular fibrillation and pulseless ventricular tachycardia (VF/VT). (Reproduced with permission from Journal of the American Medical Association: Guidelines for cardiopulmonary resuscitation and emergency cardiac care 1992, Vol. 268, CPR issue, pp 2199–2241, Copyrighted 1992, American Medical Association.)

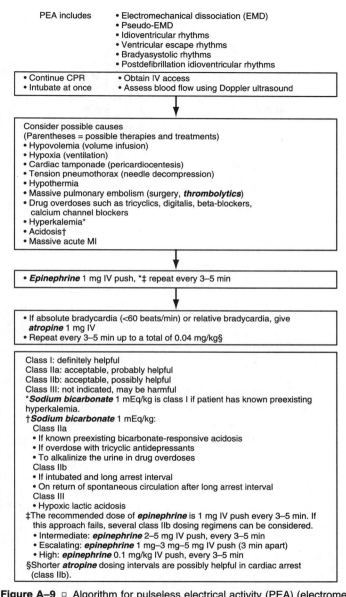

PEA includes
- Electromechanical dissociation (EMD)
- Pseudo-EMD
- Idioventricular rhythms
- Ventricular escape rhythms
- Bradyasystolic rhythms
- Postdefibrillation idioventricular rhythms

- Continue CPR
- Intubate at once
- Obtain IV access
- Assess blood flow using Doppler ultrasound

↓

Consider possible causes
(Parentheses = possible therapies and treatments)
- Hypovolemia (volume infusion)
- Hypoxia (ventilation)
- Cardiac tamponade (pericardiocentesis)
- Tension pneumothorax (needle decompression)
- Hypothermia
- Massive pulmonary embolism (surgery, *thrombolytics*)
- Drug overdoses such as tricyclics, digitalis, beta-blockers, calcium channel blockers
- Hyperkalemia*
- Acidosis†
- Massive acute MI

↓

- *Epinephrine* 1 mg IV push, *‡ repeat every 3–5 min

- If absolute bradycardia (<60 beats/min) or relative bradycardia, give *atropine* 1 mg IV
- Repeat every 3–5 min up to a total of 0.04 mg/kg§

Class I: definitely helpful
Class IIa: acceptable, probably helpful
Class IIb: acceptable, possibly helpful
Class III: not indicated, may be harmful
*_Sodium bicarbonate_ 1 mEq/kg is class I if patient has known preexisting hyperkalemia.
†*Sodium bicarbonate* 1 mEq/kg:
  Class IIa
  • If known preexisting bicarbonate-responsive acidosis
  • If overdose with tricyclic antidepressants
  • To alkalinize the urine in drug overdoses
  Class IIb
  • If intubated and long arrest interval
  • On return of spontaneous circulation after long arrest interval
  Class III
  • Hypoxic lactic acidosis
‡The recommended dose of *epinephrine* is 1 mg IV push every 3–5 min. If this approach fails, several class IIb dosing regimens can be considered.
  • Intermediate: *epinephrine* 2–5 mg IV push, every 3–5 min
  • Escalating: *epinephrine* 1 mg–3 mg–5 mg IV push (3 min apart)
  • High: *epinephrine* 0.1 mg/kg IV push, every 3–5 min
§Shorter *atropine* dosing intervals are possibly helpful in cardiac arrest (class IIb).

Figure A–9 □ Algorithm for pulseless electrical activity (PEA) (electromechanical dissociation [EMD]). (Reproduced with permission from Journal of the American Medical Association: Guidelines for cardiopulmonary resuscitation and emergency cardiac care 1992, Vol. 268, CPR issue, pp 2199–2241, Copyrighted 1992, American Medical Association.)

Figure A–10 □ Asystole treatment algorithm. (Reproduced with permission from Journal of the American Medical Association: Guidelines for cardiopulmonary resuscitation and emergency cardiac care 1992, Vol. 268, CPR issue, pp 2199–2241, Copyrighted 1992, American Medical Association.)

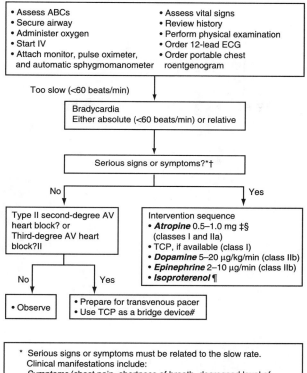

- Assess ABCs
- Secure airway
- Administer oxygen
- Start IV
- Attach monitor, pulse oximeter, and automatic sphygmomanometer

- Assess vital signs
- Review history
- Perform physical examination
- Order 12-lead ECG
- Order portable chest roentgenogram

Too slow (<60 beats/min)

Bradycardia
Either absolute (<60 beats/min) or relative

Serious signs or symptoms?*†

No   Yes

Type II second-degree AV heart block? or
Third-degree AV heart block?II

Intervention sequence
- **Atropine** 0.5–1.0 mg ‡§ (classes I and IIa)
- TCP, if available (class I)
- **Dopamine** 5–20 µg/kg/min (class IIb)
- **Epinephrine** 2–10 µg/min (class IIb)
- **Isoproterenol** ¶

No   Yes

- Observe

- Prepare for transvenous pacer
- Use TCP as a bridge device#

---

* Serious signs or symptoms must be related to the slow rate. Clinical manifestations include:
  Symptoms (chest pain, shortness of breath, decreased level of consciousness) and
  Signs (low BP, shock, pulmonary congestion, CHF, acute MI).

† Do not delay TCP while awaiting IV access or for **atropine** to take effect if patient is symptomatic.

‡ Denervated transplanted hearts will not respond to **atropine**. Go at once to pacing, **catecholamine** infusion, or both.

§ **Atropine** should be given in repeat doses in 3–5 min up to total of 0.04 mg/kg. Consider shorter dosing intervals in severe clinical conditions. It has been suggested that atropine should be used with caution in AV block at the His-Purkinje level (type II AV block and new third-degree block with wide QRS complexes) (class IIb).

II Never treat third-degree heart block plus ventricular escape beats with **lidocaine**.

¶ **Isoproterenol** should be used, if at all, with extreme caution. At low doses, it is class IIb (possibly helpful); at higher doses, it is class III (harmful).

Verify patient tolerance and mechanical capture. Use analgesia and sedation as needed.

Figure A–11 □ Bradycardia algorithm (with the patient not in cardiac arrest). (Reproduced by permission from Journal of the American Medical Association: Guidelines for cardiopulmonary resuscitation and emergency cardiac care 1992, Vol. 268, CPR issue, pp 2199–2241, Copyrighted 1992, American Medical Association.)

- Assess ABCs
- Secure airway
- Administer oxygen
- Start IV
- Attach monitor, pulse oximeter, and automatic sphygmomanometer

- Assess vital signs
- Review history
- Perform physical examination
- Order 12-lead ECG
- Order portable chest roentgenogram

Unstable, with serious signs or symptoms*

No or borderline

Yes

If ventricular rate >150 beats/min
- Prepare for immediate cardioversion (go to Fig. A–7)
- May give brief trial of medications based on arrhythmia
- Immediate cardioversion is seldom needed for heart rates <150 beats/min

---

Atrial fibrillation
Atrial flutter

Consider use of
- *Diltiazem*
- *Beta-blockers*
- *Verapamil*
- *Digoxin*
- *Procainamide*
- *Anticoagulants*

Paroxysmal supraventricular tachycardia (PSVT)

→ Vagal maneuvers†

→ • *Adenosine* 6 mg rapid IV push over 1–3 s

1-2 min →

Wide-complex tachycardia of uncertain type

→ • *Lidocaine* 1–1.5 mg/kg IV push

Every 5–10 min

→ • *Lidocaine* 0.5–0.75 mg/kg IV push, maximum total 3 mg/kg →

Ventricular tachycardia (VT)

→ • *Lidocaine* 1–1.5 mg/kg IV push

Every 5–10 min

→ • *Lidocaine* 0.5–0.75 mg/kg IV push, maximum total 3 mg/kg →

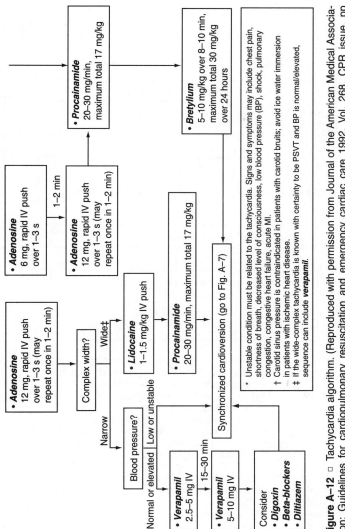

Figure A–12 □ Tachycardia algorithm. (Reproduced with permission from Journal of the American Medical Association: Guidelines for cardiopulmonary resuscitation and emergency cardiac care 1992, Vol. 268, CPR issue, pp 2199–2241, Copyrighted 1992, American Medical Association.)

* Unstable condition must be related to the tachycardia. Signs and symptoms may include chest pain, shortness of breath, decreased level of consciousness, low blood pressure (BP), shock, pulmonary congestion, congestive heart failure, acute MI.

† Carotid sinus pressure is contraindicated in patients with carotid bruits; avoid ice water immersion in patients with ischemic heart disease.

‡ If the wide-complex tachycardia is known with certainty to be PSVT and BP is normal/elevated, sequence can include *verapamil.*

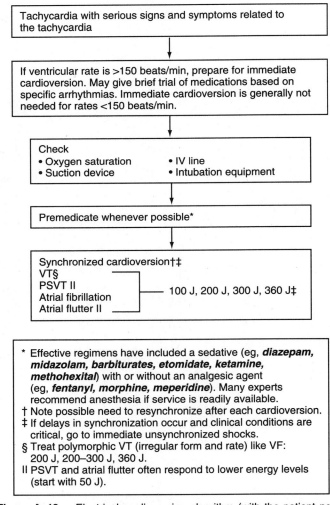

Tachycardia with serious signs and symptoms related to the tachycardia

If ventricular rate is >150 beats/min, prepare for immediate cardioversion. May give brief trial of medications based on specific arrhythmias. Immediate cardioversion is generally not needed for rates <150 beats/min.

Check
- Oxygen saturation
- Suction device
- IV line
- Intubation equipment

Premedicate whenever possible*

Synchronized cardioversion†‡
VT§
PSVT ll
Atrial fibrillation
Atrial flutter ll ─────── 100 J, 200 J, 300 J, 360 J‡

* Effective regimens have included a sedative (eg, *diazepam, midazolam, barbiturates, etomidate, ketamine, methohexital*) with or without an analgesic agent (eg, *fentanyl, morphine, meperidine*). Many experts recommend anesthesia if service is readily available.
† Note possible need to resynchronize after each cardioversion.
‡ If delays in synchronization occur and clinical conditions are critical, go to immediate unsynchronized shocks.
§ Treat polymorphic VT (irregular form and rate) like VF: 200 J, 200–300 J, 360 J.
ll PSVT and atrial flutter often respond to lower energy levels (start with 50 J).

Figure A–13 □ Electrical cardioversion algorithm (with the patient not in cardiac arrest). (Reproduced with permission from Journal of the American Medical Association: Guidelines for cardiopulmonary resuscitation and emergency cardiac care 1992, Vol. 268, CPR issue, pp 2199–2241, Copyrighted 1992, American Medical Association.)

APPENDIX B

□ □ □

ON CALL FORMULARY

This formulary includes medications that are commonly encountered while performing on call procedures. Dosages listed are for adults, and generic names are listed. Always be mindful of the renal and hepatic function of the patient prior to administration of medications, and be aware that many medications require individualization of dose. For further information, consult the pharmacy or the medication insert instructions.

ACETAMINOPHEN (Tylenol and others)   *Analgesic, antipyretic*

Indications:	Pain or fever.
Actions:	Diminishes pain response, acts directly on hypothalamic temperature-regulation centers.
Metabolism:	Hepatic.
Excretion:	Renal.
Side effects:	Uncommon—rash, drug fever, mucosal ulcerations, leukopenia, pancytopenia, and hepatic toxicity.
Dose:	325–1000 mg PO or PR q4–6h PRN, up to 4000 mg/24 h.
Notes:	Little to no anti-inflammatory action. Does not affect the aggregation of platelets. Does not interact with anticoagulants. *Antidote for overdose is N-acetylcysteine.*

ALBUTEROL (Proventil, Ventolin)   *β₂-Adrenergic agonist*

Indications:	Bronchospasm due to asthma, bronchitis, or COPD.
Actions:	β₂-Adrenergic agonist.
Metabolism:	Hepatic. Less than 20% of the inhaled dose is absorbed systemically.
Excretion:	Renal.
Side effects:	Headache, tachycardia, lightheadedness, dizziness, tremor, palpitations, nausea.
Dose:	2.5–5 mg in 3 ml NS by nebulizer q4 h PRN. Severe acute bronchospasm may require doses q3–5 min initially. Two puffs from a metered dose inhaler (MDI) q4–6 h PRN.
Notes:	May alternate with metaproterenol.

AMINOCAPROIC ACID (Amicar)   *Plasminogen activator inhibitor*

Indications:	Hemorrhage due to fibrinolysis.
Actions:	Inhibits plasminogen activator. Also has antiplasmin activity.
Metabolism:	65% of drug is excreted unchanged.
Excretion:	Renal.

Side effects:	Increased risk of DVT, cerebral embolism, and pulmonary embolism. Nausea, abdominal cramps, dizziness, rash, and headaches.
Dose:	Loading dose of 4–5 g IV over 1 h, followed by maintenance infusion of 1–1.25 g/h to achieve plasma levels of 0.13 mg/ml or until clinical bleeding stops. Maximum dose, 30 g/24 h. Loading dose may be given PO.
Notes:	Rule out DIC before administration.

AMINOPHYLLINE (Methylxanthine)   *Bronchodilator*

Indications:	Bronchospasm due to asthma.
Actions:	Inhibits phosphodiesterase activity, resulting in smooth muscle relaxation and bronchodilation. Also activates respiratory centers.
Metabolism:	Hepatic (90%).
Excretion:	Renal.
Side effects:	Tachycardia, increased ventricular ectopy, nausea, vomiting, headaches, seizures, insomnia, and nightmares.
Dose:	Loading dose of 6 mg/kg IV, followed by maintenance infusion of 0.5–0.7 mg/kg/h. Use half loading dose if the patient is already taking theophylline.
Notes:	May follow plasma level, but side effects generally limit therapeutic usefulness. Decrease the dose in patients with CHF or liver disease and in the elderly. Aminophylline clearance is decreased by erythromycin, cimetidine, propranolol, allopurinol, and a number of other medications.

ASPIRIN (Acetylsalicylic Acid)   *Analgesic, antipyretic, anti-inflammatory*

Indications:	Pain due to inflammation, fever, or antiplatelet aggregation agent in coronary syndromes.
Actions:	Acts peripherally by interfering with the production of prostaglandins, thus reducing pain and inflammation. Acts centrally to reduce pain perception and reduce temperature by increasing heat loss.
Side effects:	Gastric erosion and bleeding, tinnitus, fever, thirst, and diaphoresis. Severe allergic reactions can occur, including asthma-like symptoms.
Dose:	For mild pain or fever, 325–650 mg PO q4–6 h. For chest pain due to pericarditis, 650 mg PO QID. For angina and antiplatelet effects, 30–325 mg PO QD or every other day. For treatment of rheumatoid arthritis, 2.6–5.2 g/day in divided doses.

BECLOMETHASONE (Beclovent, Vanceril)   *Inhaled corticosteroid*

Indications:	Bronchial asthma or long-term therapy.
Actions:	Topical anti-inflammatory.
Excretion:	Fecal.
Side effects:	Oral and pharyngeal candidiasis and laryngeal myopathy.
Dose:	Two puffs from a metered dose inhaler (MDI) BID to QID. May be more effective if administered 3–5 min after a bronchodilator dose.
Notes:	Not indicated for acute bronchospasm.

BUMETANIDE (Bumex)   *Loop diuretic*

Indications: Edema associated with CHF, cirrhosis, renal disease, or nephrotic syndrome.
Actions: Inhibits the reabsorption of Na^+ and Cl^- in the ascending limb of the loop of Henle. Increases potassium excretion. Rapid onset, short duration of action.
Excretion: Renal (80%).
Side effects: Electrolyte depletion, rash, hyperuricemia, and reversible deafness.
Dose: 0.5–1.0 mg/day PO/IV in a single dose. May repeat q20 min, if necessary, to a maximum of 3 mg.
Notes: 1 mg bumetanide is equivalent to 40 mg furosemide.

CALCIUM GLUCONATE   *Calcium supplement*

Indications: Symptomatic hypocalcemia or hyperkalemia. Adjunct therapy in CPR protocol.
Actions: Replacement. Decreases cardiac automaticity, raises cardiac cell resting potential.
Side effects: Administration to patients concurrently receiving digoxin therapy may precipitate ventricular dysrhythmias due to combined effects of digoxin and Ca^{2+}.
Dose: For control of hypocalcemia, 1–15 g PO QD. For more rapid response, 5–10 ml of 10% solution IV.
Notes: 500 mg of calcium gluconate = 2.3 mmol Ca^{2+}. 10% solution contains 0.45 mmol Ca^{2+}/ml.

CAPTOPRIL (Capoten)   *Angiotensin-converting enzyme (ACE) inhibitor*

Indications: Hypertension, CHF, or prophylaxis against diabetic nephropathy.
Actions: Inhibits the enzyme responsible for pulmonary conversion of angiotensin I to angiotensin II.
Excretion: Renal (95%).
Side effects: Hypotension, impaired taste, cough, rash, angioedema, neutropenia, proteinuria, and renal insufficiency.
Dose: Begin with a test dose of 6.25 mg PO and monitor BP for 4 h. For hypertension, titrate up to 25–50 mg PO BID or TID. For CHF, titrate up to 25–50 mg PO TID.
Notes: May cause hyperkalemia if used in patients receiving potassium-sparing diuretics or potassium supplementation.

CHLORAL HYDRATE   *Hypnotic*

Indications: Insomnia.
Actions: Hypnotic.
Side effects: Gastric irritation, rash, and *paradoxical agitation*.
Dose: 0.5–1.0 g PO or PR QHS PRN.
Notes: Avoid in patients with liver or kidney disease.

CHLORDIAZEPOXIDE (Librium and others) *Benzodiazepine*

Indications: Anxiety or alcohol withdrawal.
Actions: Benzodiazepine sedative, anxiolytic agent.
Metabolism: Hepatic.
Excretion: Renal.
Side effects: CNS depression, drowsiness, ataxia, confusion, and pruritic rash.
Dose: For anxiety, 5–25 mg PO TID to QID. For alcohol withdrawal, 50–100 mg IM or IV q2–6 h PRN, maximum dose of 500 mg in the first 24 h.
Notes: Dose must be individualized. Unpredictable absorption after IM injection. *Antidote is flumazenil.*

CHLORPROMAZINE (Thorazine) *Antipsychotic phenothiazine, antiemetic*

Indications: Agitation, nausea, vomiting, or hiccoughs.
Actions: Antagonist of dopaminergic, histaminergic, muscurenergic, and α_1-adrenergic responses.
Side effects: CNS depression, hypotension, extrapyramidal effects, and jaundice.
Dose: For mild agitation, 25–75 mg PO QD. For more severe cases, 150 mg PO QD or 25–50 mg IM with repeated doses q3–4 h PRN. For hiccoughs, nausea, and vomiting, 10–25 mg PO or IM q6–8 h.
Notes: For acute agitation, haloperidol may be a more appropriate choice because it has less effect on the BP.

CIMETIDINE (Tagamet) *Histamine$_2$ antagonist*

Indications: Peptic ulcer disease or gastroesophageal reflux.
Actions: Inhibits histamine-induced secretion of gastric acid.
Metabolism: Hepatic.
Excretion: Renal.
Side effects: Gynecomastia, impotence, confusion, diarrhea, leukopenia, thrombocytopenia, and increased serum creatinine.
Dose: For peptic ulcer, 300 mg PO or IV q6–8 h, or 800 mg PO QHS. For reflux, 400 mg PO BID.
Notes: Reduces microsomal enzyme metabolism of medications, including oral anticoagulants, phenytoin, and theophylline.

CODEINE *Narcotic analgesic*

Indications: Pain, cough, or diarrhea.
Actions: Narcotic analgesic. Depresses the medullary cough center, decreases propulsive contractions of the small bowel.
Metabolism: Hepatic.
Excretion: Renal (90%).
Side effects: Dysphoria, agitation, pruritus, constipation, lightheadedness, and sedation.
Dose: For analgesia, 30–60 mg PO, SQ, or IM q4–6 h PRN. For cough or diarrhea, 8–30 mg PO, SQ, or IM q4 h PRN.
Notes: Useful for mild to moderate pain. *May be habit forming.*

DIAZEPAM (Valium and others)   *Benzodiazepine*

Indications:	Anxiety, seizures, or alcohol withdrawal.
Actions:	Benzodiazepine sedative, anxiolytic agent.
Metabolism:	Hepatic (to active metabolites).
Excretion:	Renal.
Side effects:	Sedation, hypotension, respiratory depression, and *paradoxical agitation*.
Dose:	For anxiety, 2–10 mg PO, IM, or IV BID to QID. For status epilepticus, 2 mg/min IV until the seizure ceases or to a total dose of 20 mg. For alcohol withdrawal, 5–10 mg IV at a rate of 2–5 mg/min q30–60 min until the patient is sedate, then maintain on 10–20 mg PO QID.
Notes:	Dose be individualized. Unpredictable absorption after IM injection. Rectal and ET administration routes are possible in emergency situations. *Antidote is flumazenil.*

DIGOXIN (Lanoxin)   *Digitalis glycoside*

Indications:	Supraventricular tachycardia or CHF.
Actions:	Slows AV conduction, increases the force of cardiac contraction, Na^+, K^+-ATPase inhibitor.
Metabolism:	Hepatic (<10%).
Excretion:	Renal (80%).
Side effects:	Dysrhythmias, nausea, vomiting, and neuropsychiatric disturbances.
Dose:	Load with 0.125–0.5 mg IV q6 h to a total dose of 1 mg, or load with 0.125–0.5 mg PO q6 h to a total dose of 1.5 mg, then maintain on 0.125–0.25 mg PO or IV QD. Some supraventricular tachycardias may require higher doses.
Notes:	Reduce dose in the elderly and in patients with renal impairment. May cause dysrhythmias in setting of hypokalemia or hypercalcemia.

DILTIAZEM (Cardizem, Dilacor)   *Calcium channel blocker*

Indications:	Angina pectoris, coronary spasm, or hypertension.
Actions:	Calcium channel blocker, vasodilator.
Metabolism:	Hepatic.
Excretion:	Renal and biliary.
Side effects:	First-degree AV block, bradycardia, flushing, dizziness, headache, peripheral edema, nausea, rash, and asthenia.
Dose:	Initial dose, 30 mg PO TID to QID, with titration to 180–360 mg/day administered in divided doses.
Notes:	Maximum antihypertensive effect is seen at 14 days. Sustained-release forms are available.

DIPHENHYDRAMINE (Benadryl)   *Antihistamine*

Indications:	Allergic reactions.
Actions:	Antihistamine and anticholinergic.
Metabolism:	Hepatic.
Excretion:	Renal.
Side effects:	Drowsiness, dizziness, dry mouth, and urinary retention.

Dose: 25–50 mg PO, IV, or IM q6–8 h PRN.
Notes: Anticholinergic effects may be additive to those noted
               with other medications, such as tricyclic antidepressants.

ENALAPRIL (Vasotec)   *Angiotensin-converting enzyme (ACE) inhibitor*

Indications: Hypertension or CHF.
Actions: Inhibits the enzyme responsible for conversion of angio-
               tensin I to angiotensin II.
Metabolism: Hepatic (to active metabolite, enalaprilat).
Excretion: Renal.
Side effects: Hypotension, headache, nausea, and diarrhea.
Dose: Begin with a test dose of 2.5 mg PO and monitor BP for
               4 h. For hypertension, titrate up to 2.5–40 mg PO QD.
               For CHF, titrate up to 10–25 mg PO BID.
Notes: May cause hyperkalemia if used in patients receiving
               potassium-sparing diuretics or potassium supplementa-
               tion.

ETHACRYNIC ACID (Edecrin)   *Loop diuretic*

Indications: CHF or edema.
Actions: Inhibition of the reabsorption of Na^+ and Cl^- in the
               ascending limb of the loop of Henle.
Side effects: Electrolyte depletion, hyperuricemia, hyperglycemia,
               anorexia, nausea, vomiting, diarrhea, and sensorioneu-
               ral hearing loss.
Dose: 50 mg IV for one or two doses.
Notes: May have more side effects than other loop diuretics.
               Onset is rapid, within 30 min of a PO dose or within 5
               min of an IV dose.

FAMOTIDINE (Pepcid)   *Histamine$_2$ antagonist*

Indications: Peptic ulcer disease or gastroesophageal reflux.
Actions: Inhibits histamine-induced secretion of gastric acid.
Metabolism: Hepatic (to inactive metabolite).
Excretion: Renal (70%).
Side effects: Headache, dizziness, constipation, diarrhea, GI upset,
               and rash.
Dose: For acute disease, 40 mg PO QD or 20 mg IV BID. For
               maintenance, 20 mg PO QHS.
Notes: Less effect on microsomal enzymes and less androgen
               receptor antagonism than cimetidine.

FLUMAZENIL (Romazicon)   *Benzodiazepine antagonist*

Indications: Reversal of benzodiazepine-induced sedation.
Actions: Benzodiazepine receptor antagonist.
Metabolism: Hepatic.
Excretion: Renal.
Side effects: Seizures, headache, vasodilation, nausea, vomiting, agi-
               tation, dizziness, abnormal vision, and paresthesias.
Dose: For reversal of sedation, 0.2 mg IV over 15 s. Repeat as
               necessary in increments of 0.2 mg q60 s, to a maximum
               dose of 1 mg. For treatment of benzodiazepine overdose,

0.2 mg IV over 30 s. An additional 0.3 mg IV may be administered after 30 s, if necessary. Further doses of 0.5 mg may be given IV q30 s as needed to a maximum of 3 mg.

Notes:	Avoid in patients with evidence of cyclic antidepressant overdose. Does not reverse benzodiazepine-induced respiratory depression. Monitor for return of benzodiazepine-related symptoms of sedation and respiratory depression.

FUROSEMIDE (Lasix) *Loop diuretic*

Indications:	CHF, edema, hyperkalemia, or hypercalcemia.
Actions:	Inhibition of the reabsorption of Na^+ and Cl^- in the ascending limb of the loop of Henle.
Metabolism:	Hepatic.
Excretion:	Renal.
Side effects:	Electrolyte depletion, hyperuricemia, hyperglycemia, and reversible deafness.
Dose:	For acute pulmonary edema, 20–40 mg PO or IV with repeat doses q60–90 min PRN, to a maximum of 600 mg/day. Higher doses may be required in patients with severe disease or renal failure.
Notes:	Loop diuretics are well absorbed orally with a rapid onset of action.

HALOPERIDOL (Haldol) *Antipsychotic*

Indications:	Psychotic disorders or acute agitation.
Actions:	Antipsychotic neuroleptic butyrophenone.
Side effects:	Extrapyramidal reactions, postural hypotension, sedation, galactorrhea, jaundice, blurred vision, bronchospasm, and neuroleptic malignant syndrome.
Dose:	0.5–2.0 mg PO TID. For acute psychotic crises, 2–10 mg IM q1 h PRN.
Notes:	Extrapyramidal side effects are more pronounced, but hypotension is less frequent than with phenothiazines.

HEPARIN SODIUM *Anticoagulant*

Indications:	Prophylaxis and treatment of DVT, pulmonary embolism, or embolic CVA. Adjunct in treatment of unstable angina, thrombolytic therapy.
Actions:	Acts in conjunction with anti–thrombin III, which neutralizes several activated clotting factors. Antithrombin effect.
Metabolism:	Hepatic.
Excretion:	Renal.
Side effects:	Hemorrhage and thrombocytopenia.
Dose:	For DVT or pulmonary embolus, load IV with 5000–10,000 units followed by continuous infusion of 1000–2000 units/h IV. Low-dose SQ: 5000 units q8–12 h. High-dose SQ: 10,000–12,500 units q8–12 h. Titrate to desired PTT (generally 1½–2× control).

Notes: Monitor PTT closely. Also prolongs PT. Overheparinization is treated with *protamine sulfate*. Usual dose is 1 mg protamine/100 units of heparin given slowly IV.

HYDRALAZINE (Apresoline) *Arterial vasodilator*

Indications: Hypertension.
Actions: Arterial vasodilator.
Metabolism: Hepatic.
Side effects: Tachycardia, headache, blood dyscrasias, nausea, vomiting, diarrhea, and SLE reaction at higher doses (>200 mg/day).
Dose: 10–25 mg PO q6 h. 20–40 mg IV or IM q3–6 h PRN.
Notes: Very limited effect on veins, so minimal postural hypotension. Monitor carefully in patients with coronary artery disease.

HYDROCHLOROTHIAZIDE (Esidrix HydroDIURIL) *Thiazide diuretic*

Indications: Hypertension, CHF, or edema.
Actions: Blocks Na^+ and Cl^- reabsorption in the cortical diluting segment of the loop of Henle.
Excretion: Renal.
Side effects: Electrolyte depletion, hyperuricemia, hyperglycemia, hypercalcemia, pancreatitis, jaundice, nausea, vomiting, and diarrhea.
Dose: 12.5–50 mg PO QD.
Notes: Adequate potassium replacement necessary with long-term therapy.

HYDROCORTISONE *Corticosteroid*

Indications: Severe bronchospasm, anaphylaxis, hypercalcemia, or adrenal insufficiency.
Actions: Anti-inflammatory.
Side effects: Na^+ retention, hyperglycemia, and K^+ loss. Behavioral disturbances.
Dose: 250 mg IV followed by 100 mg IV q6 h.
Notes: Contraindicated in settings of systemic fungal infections.

HYDROXYZINE (Atarax, Vistaril) *Antihistamine, antiemetic*

Indications: Anxiety, pruritus, nausea, or vomiting.
Actions: Suppression of activity in subcortical CNS sites.
Metabolism: Hepatic.
Side effects: Drowsiness, dry mouth, and tremor.
Dose: For anxiety, 50–100 mg PO or IM QID. For pruritus or nausea, 25–100 mg PO or IM TID to QID.
Notes: May potentiate the sedation effects of other CNS depressants.

IBUPROFEN (Motrin and others) *NSAID*

Indications: Inflammation due to arthritis, soft tissue injuries, or analgesia.

Actions:	Propionic acid derivative. Interferes with the production of prostaglandins.
Metabolism:	Hepatic.
Excretion:	Renal.
Side effects:	Nausea, diarrhea, gastric pain, gastric erosions, dizziness, headache, tinnitus, and vision changes. May compromise renal function in patients with renal impairment. Contraindicated in the syndrome of aspirin sensitivity, nasal polyps, and bronchospasm.
Dose:	For analgesia, 200 mg PO TID to QID. For anti-inflammatory effects, 200–400 mg PO TID to QID. Maximum dose: 3200 mg/d.
Notes:	Available in many over-the-counter preparations. Should be used with caution in patients receiving anticoagulant medications.

INDOMETHACIN (Indocin) *NSAID*

Indications:	Inflammation due to arthritis, acute gout, soft tissue injury, or pericarditis.
Actions:	Indole acetic acid derivative. Interferes with the production of prostaglandins.
Metabolism:	Hepatic.
Excretion:	Renal.
Side effects:	Headache, dizziness and lightheadedness, and epigastric pain. May compromise renal function in patients with renal impairment. Contraindicated in the syndrome of aspirin sensitivity, nasal polyps, and bronchospasm.
Dose:	25–50 mg PO TID. Maximum daily dose, 150–200 mg/d.
Notes:	May increase the risk of bleeding in patients receiving anticoagulants. Take with food to minimize GI upset.

INSULIN *Hypoglycemic*

Indications:	Diabetes mellitus.
Actions:	Enhances hepatic glycogen storage, enhances entry of glucose and potassium into cells, inhibits the breakdown of protein and fat.
Side effects:	Hypoglycemia, local skin reactions, and lipohypertrophy.
Dose:	Must be individualized.
Notes:	Less immunogenicity is seen with recombinant human insulin than with insulins from animal sources.

ISOSORBIDE DINITRATE (Isordil, Sorbitrate) *Vasodilator*

Indications:	Angina pectoris or CHF.
Actions:	Venous, coronary, and arterial vasodilator.
Side effects:	Headache, hypotension, and flushing.
Dose:	5–30 mg PO QID.
Notes:	Nitrate tolerance may develop with prolonged continuous administration.

LABETALOL (Normodyne, Trandate) *α₁- and β-blocker*

Indications:	Hypertensive emergencies.
Actions:	α_1-Blocking action is predominant in acute use but is accompanied by nonspecific β-blockade.
Metabolism:	Hepatic.
Excretion:	Renal.
Side effects:	Postural hypotension, bronchospasm, jaundice, bradycardia, and negative inotropic effect. Avoid in patients with asthma or severe bradycardia.
Dose:	20 mg IV q10–15 min. Increase the dose incrementally (e.g., 20 mg, 20 mg, 40 mg, 40 mg . . .) q10 min until the desired supine BP is achieved. Alternately, a continuous drip may be started at 2 mg/min with titration to desired BP response, with a maximum daily dose of 2400 mg.
Notes:	Contraindicated in patients in whom β-blockade is undesirable.

LIDOCAINE (Xylocaine) *Class IB antiarrhythmic*

Indications:	Ventricular arrhythmias—prophylaxis, and treatment.
Actions:	Lengthens the effective refractory period in the ventricular conduction system. Decreases ventricular automaticity.
Metabolism:	Hepatic.
Excretion:	Renal.
Side effects:	Nausea, vomiting, hypotension, confusion, seizures, perioral paresthesias, drowsiness, and dizziness.
Dose:	Load with 1 mg/kg IV over 2–3 min. Further doses of 50 mg IV may be given at 5- to 10-min intervals to a total dose of 300 mg. Maintain with 1–4 mg/min continuous IV infusion. For prophylaxis, a loading dose of 200 mg given in 50-mg increments q5 min, followed by maintenance IV infusion of 3 mg/min.
Notes:	Lower maintenance doses are required in elderly patients or in those with CHF, hepatic failure, or hypotension.

LORAZEPAM (Ativan) *Benzodiazepine*

Indications:	Insomnia or anxiety.
Actions:	Benzodiazepine sedative-hypnotic.
Metabolism:	Hepatic.
Excretion:	Renal.
Side effects:	Sedation and respiratory depression.
Dose:	For sleep, 0.5–1.0 mg PO or IM QHS. For anxiety, 1 mg PO or IM TID. Maximum dose, 4 mg/dose.
Notes:	Peak effect in 1–6 h. *Antidote is flumazenil.*

MANNITOL (Osmitrol) *Osmotic diuretic*

Indications:	Peripheral edema, cerebral edema, or hemolytic transfusion reactions.

Actions:	Osmotic diuresis.
Excretion:	Renal.
Side effects:	Volume overload, hyperosmolality, hyponatremia, nausea, and headache.
Dose:	Test dose of 12.5 g over 3–5 min. Effects should be noted within 2 h. 25–100 g IV over 15–30 min q2–3 h PRN.
Notes:	Requires functioning kidneys to work, contraindicated in renal failure. Monitor electrolytes.

MEPERIDINE (Demerol)   *Narcotic analgesic*

Indications:	Moderate to severe pain.
Actions:	Narcotic analgesic.
Metabolism:	Hepatic.
Excretion:	Renal.
Side effects:	Respiratory depression, hypotension, nausea, vomiting, constipation, agitation, and rash.
Dose:	50–150 mg SC, IM, or PO q4 h; 10–50 mg IV.
Notes:	60–80 mg meperidine (SQ, IM, or PO) is equivalent to 10 mg morphine (SC or IV). Often administered with concomitant antinausea medication. *Antidote is naloxone. May be habit forming.*

METAPROTERENOL (Alupent, Metaprel)   *β₂-Adrenergic agonist*

Indications:	Bronchospasm due to asthma, bronchitis, or COPD.
Actions:	β_2-Adrenergic agonist.
Metabolism:	Hepatic. 3% of aerosol dose is systemically absorbed.
Side effects:	Headache, tachycardia, hypertension, lightheadedness, dizziness, tremor, palpitations, nausea, and vomiting.
Dose:	0.2–0.3 mg in 3 ml NS by nebulizer q4 h PRN. Severe acute bronchospasm may require doses q3–5 min initially. Two puffs from a metered dose inhaler (MDI) q4–6 h PRN.
Notes:	May alternate with albuterol.

METOLAZONE (Zaroxolyn)   *Quinazoline diuretic*

Indications:	Hypertension, CHF, edema, or some types of renal failure.
Actions:	Blocks Na^+ and Cl^- reabsorption in the cortical diluting segment of the loop of Henle.
Excretion:	Renal.
Side effects:	Electrolyte depletion, hyperuricemia, hyperglycemia, and hypomagnesemia. Do not use in anuric patients.
Dose:	2.5–10 mg PO QD.
Notes:	Similar properties to thiazide diuretics but longer acting than hydrochlorothiazide. Monitor electrolytes. Additive effects when administered with furosemide.

MIDAZOLAM (Versed)   *Benzodiazepine*

Indications:	Sedation before surgery or diagnostic procedure.
Actions:	Benzodiazepine sedative-hypnotic.
Side effects:	Sedation, *paradoxical agitation*, and respiratory depression.

Dose:
Induction dose, 0.20–0.35 mg/kg IV PRN over 20–30 s. Reduce dose in elderly patients and in those already receiving other sedative medications.

Notes:
Inject slowly to avoid complications of respiratory depression and hypotension. Should be used with appropriate monitoring for respiratory complications. *Antidote is flumazenil.*

MORPHINE SULFATE   *Narcotic analgesic*

Indications:
Moderate to severe pain or pulmonary edema.

Actions:
Narcotic analgesia and splanchnic venodilation.

Metabolism:
Hepatic.

Excretion:
Renal (90%), biliary (7–10%).

Side effects:
Respiratory depression, hypotension, sedation, nausea, vomiting, and constipation.

Dose:
For pulmonary edema or chest pain due to coronary ischemia, 2–4 mg IV q5–10 min to a maximum dose of 10–12 mg. For pain, 2–15 mg IV, IM, or SQ q4 h PRN.

Notes:
10 mg morphine (IM or SQ) is equivalent to 60–80 mg meperidine (IM, SQ, or PO). Often administered with concomitant antinausea medication. *May be habit forming. Antidote is naloxone.*

NALOXONE HYDROCHLORIDE (Narcan)   *Narcotic antagonist*

Indications:
Reversal of narcotic-induced effects.

Actions:
Narcotic receptor antagonist.

Metabolism:
Hepatic.

Excretion:
Renal.

Side effects:
Nausea, vomiting, and may precipitate withdrawal in narcotic abusers.

Dose:
0.2–2.0 mg IV, IM, or SQ q5 min to a maximum dose of 10 mg.

Notes:
Effects are shorter than those of most narcotics. Monitor for return of narcotic-induced symptoms, and repeat naloxone dose as necessary. May be administered via ET in emergency situations.

NAPROXEN (Naprosyn)   *NSAID*

Indications:
Inflammation due to arthritis, soft tissue injury, or pericarditis.

Actions:
Propionic acid derivative. Interferes with production of prostaglandins.

Metabolism:
Hepatic.

Excretion:
Renal.

Side effects:
Headaches, dizziness and lightheadedness, and epigastric pain. May compromise renal function in patients with renal impairment. Contraindicated in the syndrome of aspirin sensitivity, nasal polyps, and bronchospasm.

Dose:
250 mg PO BID. Maximum dose, 1250 mg/d.

Notes:
Should be used with caution in patients receiving anticoagulant medications.

NIFEDIPINE (Adalat, Procardia)   *Calcium channel blocker*

Indications:	Angina pectoris, coronary spasm, or hypertension.
Actions:	Calcium channel blocker, vasodilator.
Metabolism:	Hepatic.
Excretion:	Renal (80%).
Side effects:	Hypotension, flushing, dizziness, headache, and peripheral edema.
Dose:	10–30 mg PO TID. Maximum dose, 180 mg/d.
Notes:	The edema caused by nifedipine is due to vasodilation and does not respond to diuretics. Hypotension is often difficult to treat with fluids alone and may require the administration of a vasopressor agent. Nifedipine has a greater effect than verapamil and diltiazem in peripheral vasculature.

NITROGLYCERIN   *Vasodilator*

Indications:	Angina pectoris or CHF.	
Actions:	Venous, coronary, and arterial vasodilation.	
Metabolism:	Hepatic.	
Excretion:	Renal.	
Side effects:	Headache, hypotension, and flushing.	
Dose:	*Sublingual:*	0.15–0.6 mg q3–5 min.
	Lingual aerosol:	1–2 sprays onto or under the tongue q3–5 min to a maximum dose of 3 sprays/15 min.
	Transdermal patch:	0.2 mg/h, increasing to 0.4 mg/h. Patch should be left on for 10–12 h and then removed for 12–14 h to avoid tolerance.
	Transdermal paste:	0.5–4 inches q4–8 h. Rotate sites.
	Oral (sustained release):	2–9 mg PO BID to TID.
	IV:	0–3 μg/kg/min. Titrate to desired BP.
Notes:	Nitrate tolerance may develop with prolonged continuous administration. Dose must be individualized.	

OMEPRAZOLE (Prilosec)   *H⁺, K⁺-ATPase inhibitor*

Indications:	Active peptic ulcer disease, gastroesophageal reflux, severe erosive esophagitis, or gastric acid hypersecretion.
Actions:	Gastric acid pump inhibitor.
Excretion:	Renal (77%), remainder biliary.
Side effects:	Headache, diarrhea, abdominal pain, nausea, vomiting, rash, and dizziness.

Dose: For ulcer, reflux, and esophagitis, 20 mg PO QD. For hypersecretion syndromes, start with 60 mg PO QD, and increase to 120 mg TID as required to achieve desired results.

Notes: Not recommended for long-term maintenance therapy.

OXAZEPAM (Serax) *Benzodiazepine*

Indications: Insomnia or anxiety.
Actions: Benzodiazepine sedative-hypnotic.
Side effects: Sedation, respiratory depression, and confusion.
Dose: For sleep, 10–30 mg PO QHS PRN. For anxiety, 30–100 mg PO QD in divided doses.
Notes: Peak effect in 1–4 h. Relatively short duration. *Antidote is flumazenil.*

PHENAZOPYRIDINE (Pyridium) *Urinary analgesic*

Indications: Cystitis or urethritis.
Actions: Analgesic effect on inflamed urinary tract mucosa.
Excretion: Renal.
Side effects: Orange discoloration of secretions including urine, tears, and semen. Nausea, headache, rash, and pruritus.
Dose: 200 mg PO TID after meals, PRN.
Notes: No antibacterial effects. May stain contact lenses.

PHENYTOIN (Dilantin) *Anticonvulsant*

Indications: Seizure disorders—prophylaxis and treatment.
Actions: Anticonvulsant, reduces Na^+ transport across cerebral cell membranes.
Metabolism: At therapeutic doses, phenytoin is metabolized by the liver in zero-order kinetics (a fixed amount of drug is metabolized per unit of time). Relatively small changes in the dose can cause major changes in serum concentrations of the long term. Serum levels are greatly affected by medications that alter microsomal enzyme activity.
Excretion: Renal.
Side effects: Hypotension, cardiac dysrhythmias, ataxia, nystagmus, dysarthria, hepatotoxicity, gingival hypertrophy, hirsutism, megaloblastic anemia, lymphadenopathy, fever, and rash.
Dose: For status epilepticus, 18 mg/kg IV in NS loading dose at a rate of 25–50 mg/min, followed by a maintenance dose of 300 mg PO or IV QD.
Notes: Dose must be individualized. Follow serum levels. IM administration is erratically absorbed. Abrupt withdrawal may precipitate seizure activity.

PHYTONADIONE (Vitamin K₁) (AquaMEPHYTON) *Vitamin replacement*

Indications: Replacement in vitamin K deficiency or reversal of warfarin effects.
Actions: Vitamin K is essential for hepatic synthesis of clotting factors II, VII, IX, and X.

Side effects:	Hematoma formation with SQ or IM administration.
Dose:	For reversal of overcoumarization, 2.5–5.0 mg PO/SQ, or IM. For vitamin supplementation in TPN, 2–5 mg IM weekly.
Notes:	Avoid IV administration because of hypotension and anaphylaxis. Severe hemorrhage due to warfarin therapy is best treated with fresh frozen plasma. The effects of vitamin K take several days to overcome with continuous warfarin therapy.

POTASSIUM (Slow-K, Micro-K, Kay Ciel)   *Potassium supplement*

Indications:	Hypokalemia.
Actions:	Potassium supplement.
Side effects:	Nausea, vomiting, diarrhea, abdominal discomfort, and hyperkalemia.
Dose:	For prevention, 24–40 mEq/day. For treatment, 60–120 mEq/day.
Notes:	Danger of hyperkalemia in patients with renal impairment or patients receiving potassium-sparing diuretics or angiotensin-converting enzyme (ACE) inhibitors.

PROCAINAMIDE (Procanbid)   *Class IA anti-arrhythmic*

Indications:	Atrial and ventricular dysrhythmias.
Actions:	Reduces the maximum rate of depolarization in atrial and ventricular conducting tissue.
Metabolism:	Hepatic.
Excretion:	Renal.
Side effects:	Hypotension, anorexia, nausea, vomiting, heart block, dysrhythmia, rash, fever, SLE-like syndrome, and arthralgias.
Dose:	Load with 1 g PO followed by 250–500 mg PO q3 h. Delayed-release formulations may be given q12 h. For life-threatening dysrhythmias, 100 mg IV over 2 min, repeat the dose until the dysrhythmia abates to a maximum dose of 1 g. Follow with a maintenance infusion of 2–4 mg/min.
Notes:	Actions are similar to quinidine except there is no atropinic effect. Cross-allergic with procaine.

PROCHLORPERAZINE (Compazine)   *Phenothiazine*

Indications:	Agitation, nausea, or vomiting.
Actions:	Antagonist of dopaminergic, histaminergic, muscurenergic, and α_1-adrenergic responses.
Metabolism:	Hepatic, with enterohepatic recirculation.
Excretion:	Renal.
Side effects:	Drowsiness, dizziness, amenorrhea, blurred vision, skin reactions, hypotension, extrapyramidal effects, jaundice, tardive dyskinesia, and neuroleptic malignant syndrome.
Dose:	For nausea, 5–10 mg PO or IM q6–8 h PRN or 2.5–10 mg IV q6–8 h PRN.

Notes: Extrapyramidal symptoms may be treated with *diphenhydramine*.

PROMETHAZINE (Phenergan) *Phenothiazine*

Indications: Sedation, antianxiety, nausea, or vomiting.
Actions: Antihistamine and anticholinergic.
Metabolism: Hepatic.
Excretion: Renal, fecal.
Side effects: Extrapyramidal symptoms, drowsiness, dizziness, constipation, dry mouth, and urinary retention.
Dose: 25–50 mg PO, PR or IM q4–6 h PRN. 12.5–25 mg IV q4–6 h PRN. Decrease dose in elderly.
Notes: Anticholinergic effects are additive with those of other medications, such as tricyclic antidepressants.

PROPRANOLOL (Inderal) *Nonspecific β-blocker*

Indications: Angina pectoris, post-MI treatment of SVT, hypertension, or thyrotoxicosis.
Actions: Nonspecific β-blockade.
Metabolism: Hepatic.
Excretion: Renal (<1%).
Side effects: Hypotension, bradycardia, bronchospasm, CHF, nausea, vomiting, fatigue, or nightmares. May mask the symptoms of hypoglycemia.
Dose: 10–80 mg PO BID to QID. Begin with a low dose and adjust to desired effect.
Notes: Abrupt withdrawal may precipitate symptoms of angina in patients with coronary artery disease. Dose must be individualized.

PROTAMINE SULFATE *Heparin antagonist*

Indications: Reversal of heparin-induced anticoagulation.
Actions: Binds to and inactivates heparin.
Side effects: Hypotension, bradycardia, and flushing.
Dose: 1 mg/100 mg heparin. Administer by slow IV push, no more than 50 mg in a 10-min period.
Notes: Overdose may paradoxically worsen hemorrhage because protamine also possesses anticoagulant properties. Effects may be transient.

RANITIDINE (Zantac) *Histamine$_2$ antagonist*

Indications: Peptic ulcer disease or gastroesophageal reflux.
Actions: Inhibits histamine-induced secretion of gastric acid.
Metabolism: Hepatic.
Excretion: Renal (30% of PO dose, 70% of IV dose).
Side effects: Jaundice, gynecomastia, headache, confusion, and leukopenia.
Dose: For acute symptoms, 50 mg IV q8 h or 150 mg PO BID or 300 mg PO QHS. For maintenance therapy, 150 mg PO QHS.

Notes: Generally well tolerated. Does not have the same effect
                    as cimetidine on microsomal enzymes and androgen
                    receptor antagonism.

SODIUM POLYSTYRENE SULFONATE (Kayexalate)
Cation exchange resin

Indications: Hyperkalemia.
Actions: Nonabsorbable cation exchange resin.
Side effects: Nausea, vomiting, gastric irritation, and sodium reten-
                    tion.
Dose: 15–30 g in 50–100 ml NS or 20% sorbitol PO q3–4 h or
                    50 g in 200 ml 20% sorbitol of $D_{20}W$ PR by retention
                    enema for 30–60 min.
Notes: 20 mEq Na^+ is exchanged for 20 mEq K^+ for each 15 g
                    resin given PO. Mg^{2+} and Ca^{2+} may also be exchanged.
                    Actual results are highly variable.

SPIRONOLACTONE (Aldactone)   *Aldosterone antagonist, diuretic*

Indications: Ascites, edema, hypertension, or hyperaldosteronism.
Actions: Aldosterone antagonist.
Metabolism: Hepatic (into many active metabolites).
Excretion: Renal > biliary.
Side effects: Hyponatremia, gynecomastia, confusion, and headache.
Dose: 50–100 mg/day PO (may be divided into QID dosing
                    as desired). Higher doses may be required in states of
                    hyperaldosteronism.
Notes: Most effective in states of hyperaldosteronism; however,
                    equipotent to thiazide diuretics in the treatment of hy-
                    pertension.

SUCRALFATE (Carafate)   *Sulfated disaccharide*

Indications: Peptic ulcer disease, prophylaxis and treatment.
Actions: Formation of an ulcer-adherent complex that acts as a
                    barrier to damage from gastric acid, bile salts, and pep-
                    sin. Minimal antacid properties.
Excretion: Fecal, not absorbed.
Side effects: Side effects are rare—constipation, nausea, gastric dis-
                    comfort, pruritus, rash, dizziness, headache, insomnia,
                    or vertigo.
Dose: 1 g PO QID.
Notes: May reduce the absorption and effects of many medica-
                    tions, including cimetidine, ciprofloxacin, digoxin, keto-
                    conazole, norfloxacin, phenytoin, ranitidine, tetracyc-
                    line, and theophylline. Sucralfate binds and sequesters
                    aluminum. Use with caution in renally impaired pa-
                    tients.

SUMATRIPTAN SUCCINATE (Imitrex)   *Intermittent treatment of migraine*

Indications:
Actions: Selective 5-hydroxytryptamine–like receptor agonist.
                    Causes vasoconstriction, particularly of the dilated ca-
                    rotid circulation in migraine disorder.

Side effects:	May cause coronary artery spasm. Contraindicated in patients with coronary artery disease, concomitant use of ergot alkaloid medication, concomitant use of monoamine oxidase inhibitors, uncontrolled hypertension, or hemiplegic migraine disorder. Flushing, dizziness, feelings of heat, pressure, malaise, fatigue, drowsiness, nausea, and vomiting.
Dose:	6 mg SQ or 100 mg PO. If initial dose is partially or completely successful, may repeat doses with an additional 6 mg SQ or 100 mg. Do not exceed a maximum daily PO dose of 300 mg. Do not repeat if initial dose has no effect.
Notes:	Peak effect in 15 min with SQ dose and in 0.5–5 h with PO dose.

VERAPAMIL (Isoptin, Calan) *Calcium channel blocker*

Indications:	Angina pectoris, treatment of SVTs, hypertension, or left ventricular diastolic dysfunction.
Actions:	Calcium channel blockade, depresses AV conduction.
Metabolism:	Hepatic.
Excretion:	Renal (70%), fecal.
Side effects:	CHF, bradycardia, hypotension, headache, dizziness, and constipation.
Dose:	For angina and hypertension, 80–120 mg PO TID. For SVT, 5–10 mg IV. IV administration should only occur in monitored patients.
Notes:	Calcium gluconate 1–2 g IV may reverse the negative inotropic and hypotensive effects but not the AV block.

WARFARIN (Coumadin) *Oral anticoagulant*

Indications:	Prophylaxis and treatment or DVT, pulmonary embolism, or embolic CVA.
Actions:	Inhibits vitamin K–dependent clotting factors.
Metabolism:	Hepatic, microsomal.
Excretion:	Renal.
Side effects:	Hemorrhage, nausea, vomiting, skin necrosis, fever, and rash.
Dose:	10 mg PO QD for 2 days, then estimate maintenance dose at 5–7.5 mg QD PO based on PT.
Notes:	Dosage must be individualized to maintain PT in the desired range. Many medications interact to increase or decrease the effects of warfarin. Always look up the interactions with warfarin of any newly prescribed medication. Fresh frozen plasma is the treatment of choice to reverse warfarin-associated hemorrhage. Vitamin K is used if further warfarin therapy is not desired.

INDEX

Page numbers in *italics* denote figures; page numbers
followed by t denote tables